'Everyone notices other people's nonverbal behavior, but it takes a special skill to *really see* what another person's body is doing, and how that relates to their bodily and psychological functioning. The genius of Jeremy Krauss's book is that he shows how this can be done. His expertise is amazing, as is his ability to explain it for readers whether they are parents, teachers, or therapists.'

Judith A. Hall, PhD, *University Distinguished Professor of Psychology, Emerita, Northeastern University, Boston*

'Grounded in decades of experience and embedded in contemporary neuroscience, Jeremy Krauss's book presents a transformative movement-based methodology and a compassionate perspective on motor development in children with special needs. Shifting the focus from deficits to abilities, it presents practical strategies that draw on insights into neuroplasticity and critical developmental periods, while emphasizing each child's individual skill set. Prioritizing careful observation, attuned connection, and growth through iterative learning, Krauss shows how building confidence in motor coordination enables children to engage more fully with their social environments, supporting emotional regulation, motivation, and cognitive development. Rich in case studies and images, this deeply encouraging work is an invaluable resource for clinicians, educators, families, as well as an inspiration for developmental neuroscientists.'

Stephanie Rudolph, PhD, *Assistant Professor, Albert Einstein College of Medicine*

'Developed by the author over decades of clinical work, the Jeremy Krauss Approach JKA uses touch and movement to access brain plasticity, fostering learning and growth in children with developmental challenges. Krauss's book elucidates his revolutionary and comprehensive approach and clearly teaches readers—parents, therapists, physicians, teachers, and caregivers— how to observe ability and facilitate each child's next stage of development, enabling the child to reach their full potential. I highly recommend *Fostering Potential in Children with Special Needs* to anyone interested in helping special needs children.'

Mercedes von Deck, MD, *Orthopedic Surgeon, Guild Certified Feldenkrais Practitioner, JKA practitioner*

'In *Fostering Potential in Children with Special Needs: An Abilities-Oriented Perspective on Early Childhood Motor Development*, Jeremy Krauss shares in an interesting, clear manner his compassionate and comprehensive approach to working with children who have special needs. He illuminates this process by engaging movement, touch, voice, mindfulness, and relationship. Jeremy begins with respect, acceptance, and trust in each child and their ability to become more freely who they actually are and to uncover their physical, emotional, and behavioral innate potentials. Based upon over 40 years of experience learning from each child their specific challenges and gifts, Jeremy has developed a unique and transformative practice to guide the children and to teach the adults who care deeply about them. If you have a child with special needs or engage with them in your life, "miracle moments" can bring you the joy of discovering a path of deep healing, not only for the children, but for your relationship with them. This book can inspire you.'

Bonnie Bainbridge Cohen, *author of* Basic Neurocellular Patterns: Exploring Developmental Movement

'In recent years, the importance given to early intervention in childhood has been increasing. In particular, detailed studies on neural plasticity and motor development theories have been revealed in many studies that are effective in minimizing neuromusculoskeletal problems that may occur in the later stages of life. In particular, a detailed understanding of typical and atypical motor development has become more valuable. It has been shown that motor development does not only consist of gross motor milestones such as head control, rolling, crawling, sitting, and walking, but especially the movement components and experiences performed by the baby/ child among these developmental milestones are much more effective in acquiring these skills. For this reason, it has been more clearly understood that it is essential for professionals and families to create environments where they can concentrate on these movement details, and for the child to be exposed to these experiences through trial and error. During my nearly 25 years of clinical and academic career, as a physiotherapist, I have gained a lot of experience in the approach to baby and child, and I have received and continue to receive many trainings to practice my profession better, effectively and up-to-date. One of the methods that I have taken recently and contributed to my point of view is the Jeremy Krauss Approach. As a child physiotherapist, although I know the typical nand atypical motor development in detail, I think that with this method, I understand how effective it is to observe the movement in detail, and then to experience and feel it on myself, in terms of understanding typical motor development, and then implementing to babies and children. Therefore, after learning the Jeremy Krauss Approach, I think that neurological problems are not the only reason behind the inability of the baby and/or child with special needs to perform a movement; in fact, it may be due to the limitations in experiencing movements in line with their existing potential. The Jeremy Krauss Approach has been an important and promising resource for me to fill the gap in understanding the typical and atypical motor development in children with special needs in detail from my daily practice. From this point of view, I believe that this book will be an important resource for professionals and families working with children with special needs. I sincerely congratulate Jeremy Krauss for his successful work and thank him for his field contributions.'

Bulent Elbasan, PT, PhD, *Prof. Decan at the Faculty of Health Sciences, Gazi University, and Lecturer at the Department of Physiotherapy and Rehabilitation*

'In his book *Fostering Potential in Children with Special Needs: An Abilities-Oriented Perspective on Early Childhood Motor Development*, Jeremy shares about our possibilities to flourish in adverse circumstances. He invites a way to look for the emergence of the new in every child, no matter their challenges. By meeting them from a place of acknowledging their wholeness and possibility, his sophisticated hands become a child's best friend, leading them to experience and strengthen their abilities. To support a child's journey through a sequence of allowing them to recognize "Yes, I am able" is much more than looking at the cup as half full. His method teaches us to see each child as already complete and functioning. He speaks to a quality of connection every child deserves, is waiting for, and depends on us to offer to them. It allows children to connect with their natural life force, which runs through each of us, and is often stronger in our early years of life. Jeremy wisely nudges us away from our false perceptions, full of assumptions and projections, to open ourselves to the big and small miracles unfolding in front of our eyes. Through his practice, he knows and also shows that ongoing discovery and development are genuinely possible. As a somatic therapist, I know that when parents who feel powerless meet therapists who feel hopeless, children take the toll. There is nothing more beautiful than seeing a child thrive. Let's all be inspired by Jeremy to look at special needs children with fresh eyes, learn with them, and enjoy their unique growth.'

Ale Duarte, *Teacher, Therapist, and Creator of Tune in to Children*

Fostering Potential in Children with Special Needs

An innovative contribution to therapeutic practice, *Fostering Potential in Children with Special Needs* provides a comprehensive introduction to the Jeremy Krauss Approach JKA. Building on the teachings of Dr. Moshe Feldenkrais and informed by decades of clinical work, the JKA methodology integrates expressive movement therapy, emotional regulation, and physical development, guiding readers toward a more inclusive and abilities-oriented form of practice when working with children experiencing difficulties in neurological, musculoskeletal, psychological, or socio-emotional domains.

Firmly grounded in practical application, the JKA methodology emphasizes close observation and understanding of developmentally relevant movement sequences and individual patterns, focusing on the dynamic aspects of transitional movements and positions. Rather than concentrating solely on limitations or deficits, the approach recognizes each child's individual abilities, supporting their unique developmental potential. This book contributes significantly to disability studies by reframing how practitioners perceive and support children with developmental challenges.

By shifting the paradigm from disability to ability, this book fills critical gaps in the understanding of child development and therapeutic approaches. Empowering readers with observational frameworks and practical techniques, this book is an invaluable resource for physical therapists, occupational therapists, developmental specialists, special educators, and parents.

Jeremy Krauss is an educational director and clinician who has taught internationally for over 40 years. Jeremy developed the Jeremy Krauss Approach JKA for movement-based therapeutic learning with adults and children with special needs.

Fostering Potential in Children with Special Needs

An Abilities-Oriented Perspective on Early Childhood Motor Development

JEREMY KRAUSS

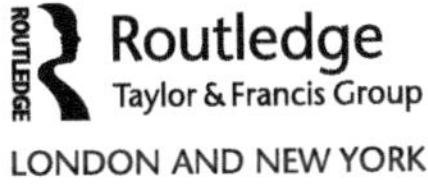

LONDON AND NEW YORK

Designed cover image: © Getty Images

First published in English 2027
by Routledge
4 Park Square, Milton Park, Abingdon, Oxon OX14 4RN

and by Routledge
605 Third Avenue, New York, NY 10158

Routledge is an imprint of the Taylor & Francis Group, an informa business

Published in German by Hogrefe 2023

British Library Cataloguing-in-Publication Data
A catalogue record for this book is available from the British Library

ISBN: 978-1-041-23763-1 (hbk)
ISBN: 978-1-041-23555-2 (pbk)
ISBN: 978-1-003-73798-8 (ebk)

DOI: 10.4324/9781003737988

Typeset in Dante and Avenir
by KnowledgeWorks Global Ltd.

To all those who seek out new perspectives and practical means to help others.

Contents

Contents

List of illustrations

Foreword
Gerald Hüther

Ever more frequently I encounter exceptionally gifted parents, pedagogues, and therapists who do a very remarkable job in supporting children.

They succeed in helping the children entrusted to them to unfold their intrinsic potential and to develop their individual possibilities in a way which outsiders might call impressive and even amazing.

More often than not, rather than taking on the support of so-called 'normal children' on their life journey, these individuals tend to focus on children who arrived into this world with some properties which make them very special.

Most of these children have more or less distinct impairments in the form of certain functional idiosyncrasies, which even the most intensive training or practice cannot convert into 'normal' versions of themselves.

The talented companions described above seem to be aware of this. So they empathize with the child and try to find what type of support this individual needs.

Accordingly, they refrain from making the child an object of their own expectations and ideas, their instructions, approaches, and treatments—something that happens all too easily. And they certainly never judge the child.

They leave it to the child to figure out for themselves how things might work, offering empathic and competent support if the child's initial attempts don't turn out so well.

In other words, they provide children with the opportunity to experience themselves as the engineers of their own learning process, as both the subjects and the designers of their own intentions and goals.

This is what makes a real difference and enables the 'miracle moments' described by Jeremy Krauss in this book to emerge: an experience of self-agency—almost impossible to express in words—of the child having accomplished something they wanted to do, which nobody would have thought possible, not even the child themselves. These are magical moments in the child's life, moments which open the door to the next developmental steps that the child will then approach with even more courage and determination—a door which otherwise would have remained shut.

This is what Moshe Feldenkrais already recognized half a century ago, and it is a phenomenon also understood by highly empathic parents, teachers, and therapists. It is very fortunate and demonstrates the growing understanding of the function and structure of the human brain that in the meantime neurobiology, too, has found ways to describe and explain the theoretical underpinnings of situations when developmental leaps of this kind occur.

But what is a theory good for if it is not put to use? How this can actually work and what kind of basic attitude it requires is shown impressively by Jeremy Krauss in his book.

Gerald Hüther, Dr. rer. nat. Dr. med. habil.,
Neurobiology, Head of the Academy for Potential Development

Preface

Working with people and especially with atypically developing special needs children is both demanding and inspiring. Daily, I encounter extraordinarily heroic children who display the best of the human spirit; children with courage and a strong desire to take part in more of life and what it has to offer.

I meet families who come to me to help their children find ways to learn, grow, and develop. Many are already resigned to a future with their child that is not promising, believing that progress and real change will take a very long time or may never come. Others are in a highly stressed state, expecting to hear yet another expert's pessimistic report on their child's future. Some come wanting to get an understanding of why their child cannot move in the same way as one of their other children. They tell me, 'My child cannot do this,' 'My child cannot do that.' The words 'cannot,' 'does not,' 'never has,' and 'will never' ring out in my practice day in, day out.

When I look at a child, I never see a child who 'cannot,' 'does not,' or 'will never.' I always look for and see a child who 'can do,' a child who 'does,' and a child 'who will.' I see a child with *potential* waiting to be tapped, with hidden abilities—a child who is searching for a possibility to emerge and grow.

My approach is an optimistic way to look at and work with the challenges and difficulties that arise in human development. It relies on accessing the brain's innate abilities to create new connections for learning, growth, and progress. Modern science unceasingly continues to unveil extraordinary processes that enable us to improve and become 'more human,' realize more potential and ability.

The brain is a wondrous biological phenomenon, which reveals to scientists, professionals, and lay people ever more astonishing and unexpected avenues to change and create better realities. The results come faster than ever thought possible. What was inconceivable becomes achievable. Change, growth, and development become the new normal. Timelines take on new meaning and are redefined. Hope and optimism evict pessimism. Satisfaction in seeing the next new step in progress takes the place of worrying whether long-term goals will ever be reached.

CASE EXAMPLE AMY

This was Amy's first visit to me. When starting a series of sessions with a child, I ask the parents about their interests and what they expect from the sessions, and how they want me to try to help their child. This day was no different. After Amy's mother had recounted her history and spoken about her genetic mutation, she said she hoped that one day Amy would be able to hold her head up while lying on her stomach and look at someone entering the room, with the top of her head to the ceiling and her eyes looking forward, and be able to tolerate this position for a few seconds. She said somberly that they had been working on it for months, with little change or improvement, but hoped that one day it would come and slowly improve. I looked closely at Amy and saw no reason why this should not be possible during the session. After establishing good contact with Amy, letting her get to know my hands and feel safe with me, I began suggesting a few directions of movements to her, to sense her responses. Amy was pleasant to be with, and with my guidance, rolled easily onto her stomach. A few moments later, after bringing both of Amy's hands into a particular arrangement, I could see what was specifically needed for her unique organization; her head quickly came up, directly and with no hesitation, all the way to vertical, with Amy supporting herself high up off her chest. She opened her eyes wide and had a precious, beaming smile on her face. She was clearly pleased to have her head up so high and was looking around with an expression of curiosity. Amy's mother was also beaming. 'How wonderful! How did you do that? She has never been able to do that before, and she looks so happy!' It was a special moment experienced and shared by all three of us.

There are moments that are extraordinary; moments that seemed unimaginable only a few seconds previously. These are moments that change not only our reality, but also the landscape of our perceptions that had seemed so impermeable. These are what I call 'miracle moments'—the moments in life that reaffirm dreams, foster optimism, and keep hope alive; the moments that bring the spirit to life within us and release the overwhelming emotions that reconnect us to the stream of life. These are the moments when the life force breaks through and appears before us. For children, miracle moments are the ones that light up their eyes and give them confidence and self-assurance. A child's entire self takes on a fresh look, and a feeling comes over them that says, 'Yes—I am able.' Miracle moments give strength and a forward-looking desire to seek and experience more such distinctive moments. Stringing moments like these together creates a continuum and a flow of unlimited directions for progress in the abilities of life.

Each and every day my work is filled with miracle moments; they are nothing out of the ordinary. Yet in the instant they appear, I am always attentive to and in awe of every miracle and the experience for all those present. I never take miracle moments for granted. I work tirelessly to pull back the screen of normalcy and enable more of these moments to emerge and be seen and experienced by others.

- 'Aha!'
- 'Wow! I can't believe she just did that!'
- 'That was amazing—he's never done that before!'
- 'She just actually did it—how did that happen?!'
- The tears of joy and pride
- The heartwarming look in a parent's eyes

These are just some of the spontaneous expressions of joy of those present during these moments. They are indeed very precious and special moments. I am always honored to be present with a parent and child when they occur. These priceless moments realize the promises of optimism and positivity, and give life a deeper meaning.

For the past 40 years, I have taught movement as therapeutic learning to thousands of children and adults—to help them improve and overcome the challenges they face every day—based on a specific way of studying movement created by Dr. Moshe Feldenkrais. Over the past 15 years, I have shifted the major focus of my work and teaching into the realm of early developmental movement and creating new and unique ways of working with special needs children. This direction of work uses ideas that delve into the most fascinating and complex area of science and understanding—the human brain and its potential. In recent decades there has been an explosion of new understanding about how our brain and nervous system develop and function, and the relationship to early motor development. This, in turn, has opened enormous vistas of comprehension regarding the potential for learning and growth at all stages of life, no matter what the conditions.

This book is about a new perspective on the development of movement and an effective way to apply this perspective to working with special needs and typically developing children, as well as to working with typically functioning adults. I have dedicated myself to educating others in this new approach that puts into practice ideas which help to achieve profound changes in children with developmental challenges, as well as in adults with functional challenges and difficulties. The perspective encompasses an optimistic and encouraging view of human potential and ability.

Laced with the practical theories of my work and stories of the children I have helped, the book also presents examples of experiential movement explorations for the reader to try out.

The book is intended to help disseminate these ideas to a wider audience and bring optimism and hope of a brighter future to children in need and their families. It is for my students, who have asked me time and time again to put my ideas into a form that they can refer back to, and for others who cannot come to study with me personally but wish to learn about my way of thinking. It is for professionals in the fields of movement, learning, and rehabilitation. It is for those interested in knowing how to realize changes previously thought unattainable. It is for therapists working with children and others interested in learning how to implement new practical ideas and applications. It is also for adults, providing more possibilities for solving functional troubles they encounter for which they still lack satisfying solutions.

In sharing my ideas now, the book which has evolved is not about techniques; it is not a how-to book or a nine-step recipe for success. It is about the ideas and concepts behind my work that allow the techniques and practical methods to come into the foreground. It presents a way of thinking about practice which enables practical applications to precipitate miracle moments. It sheds light on what to many seems vague, unclear, and often mysterious.

Acknowledgments

Many people have been generous and kind to me during the writing and development of this book, without whom it would never have been possible.

First and foremost, my heartfelt gratitude to all the special needs children and their families who never cease to inspire me and from whom I have learned so much about the wonders of the developmental process. Thanks to all the parents who kindly let me photograph their children to educate others in this important work.

To my dear wife Stephanie, a special thanks for her patience, encouragement, and support while I was writing, for reading early drafts, and for giving me honest and clear feedback. Without her, there would be no book.

To my children, Maayan, Assaf, Shani, and Livia, who inspired me from day one of each of their lives. I was able to observe each of them so closely, how they grew and developed so distinctly. Each contributed to the ideas and raw material upon which my work and this book are based.

Sabine Pfeffer for being such a good friend, colleague, and listener, always available to answer my questions, and her husband Jean-Etienne Cohen-Seat for his encouragement and guidance in so many aspects during all stages of my writing and publishing.

My brother Dr. Baruch Krauss for his very constructive, clear critique and advice during different stages of the book's development.

Livia Calice for reading all the different sections of the manuscript drafts and offering much-needed feedback.

Thanks to Dr. Sally Aldenhoven for her invaluable English editing and clarifications and for her support throughout the project from its early stages through to completion.

Gabriela Erlacher for her wonderful work on the graphics for the photo series.

A very big thank you to Lauren Redhead for her encouraging, generous support and feedback for developing the current version, as well as to Tanishka Luhia and all others at Routledge Taylor & Francis for their dedicated work.

To Hogrefe for publishing the German version of the book, particularly Susanne Ristea for pointing me in the direction needed to complete the manuscript and to Christina Nurawar Sani for her interest in my work and insightful editing collaboration.

Thanks to Dr. Alan Wiengrad, who is sadly no longer with us. Alan believed in my work early on and emphasized the importance of me putting my ideas and understanding to paper, enabling them to be shared with others and applied in a broad way.

Lastly, to my late father, who taught me in so many ways about the manifold aspects of life and its mysteries; how to listen to that which is so often not heard; how to look for and see that which most people pay no attention; how to appreciate the smallest things in life and look with daily amazement at the many of wonders that surround us but often go unnoticed.

Learning to see a child in motion   1

The starting point of the Jeremy Krauss Approach JKA is to learn to see how a child moves. This conscious observation of movement sequences includes

1. observing (visual),
2. describing (verbally, in written form), and
3. reproducing (movement).

During this unbiased watching and observing, one's attention must be actively directed toward

- individual elements,
- combinations of elements, and
- patterns.

1.1   The beginnings: my path to the Jeremy Krauss Approach JKA

When I first started working with children, I understood early on that what I saw in a typically or atypically developing child in motion was very different from that which my colleagues, students, and other people saw. When I worked with a child, observers would ask, 'What are you looking at?,' 'How do you see that?,' or 'How did you know you needed to focus on that?' I would get questions such as, 'Are you sure the child did that?,' 'When did that happen?,' 'Why is it important?' These questions seemed very peculiar

DOI: 10.4324/9781003737988-1

at the time, because it all seemed so clear to me. Was it not self-evident that when someone was watching me work with a child, that they were seeing the movements of the child as I did? Yet, gradually, I realized that not only did others *not* see what I saw, but neither could they understand what I was doing with the child or why.

One day is fixed very clearly in my memory. After a demonstration session with a special needs child, a very close colleague asked me, 'Jeremy, what you are doing looks amazing, but what exactly are you doing? What are you looking at? How do you know what to do to achieve such a clear result and an outcome that brings about such change?' I was completely puzzled. I'd never thought much about what I was doing; I'd assumed it was obvious for anyone to see. This prompted me to think about how I could help others to see the things I was seeing. Only in this way did it seem possible to share with others not only that which I was seeing, but also how and why I decided to do what I did when working with a child. I needed to find a way to teach and show others how I was able to produce such extra-ordinary changes so specifically and quickly. These changes that amazed my students and the help-seeking parents are the kinds of changes that I later describe as *moments of experience* (see Chapter 5.5), the moments in which miracles take place. It dawned on me that my manner of teaching up until this point had clearly been insufficient. I needed to devise an entirely new method of teaching, approaching, and presenting the ideas and knowledge I possessed in a way that would allow and lead others to discover for themselves how to clearly see a child in motion. Without an entirely new pedagogical and practical approach, my work and understanding would remain mine alone.

There are four key elements to studying and learning my approach: *observation*, *description*, *doing*, and *applying*. Each element is essential, and all four combined create a highly potent learning tool. It is important to learn how to see *specifically* what you are actually looking at in a child who is in motion. Think for a moment of what it is like to watch a typically developing 9- to 11-month-old child move around for one minute or so. How many and what kinds of movements does the child perform while you are watching? This may seem like an easy task, but to really appreciate how many detailed and skilled movements the child actually carries out, try to imagine that immediately after watching the baby, you must write detailed notes on all the movements, including the transitions, positions, and fine adjustments, that the child performed during this minute. How long would it take you? Could you describe them all? How quickly did the movements pass you by? Would you want or need to see it again in order to remember everything? How many movements could you remember and describe in specific detail? Some may think that one minute or so is not a long time; however, if you actually tried to write down in detail all the movements a child enacts during one minute, you would be astounded.

1.2   A new model of self-learning

The process of self-discovery and experiential learning through movement was part of the basic education provided to me personally by Dr. Moshe Feldenkrais. In this particular type of self-learning, Dr. Feldenkrais considered it essential that the learning not be based on any kind of outside image (Feldenkrais, 1972): it was to be arrived at through verbal cues. These verbal cues must be converted into sensorimotor action by their recipient, without any external model of comparison. It is a type of heuristic mode of learning using movement as the medium.

The idea of Dr. Feldenkrais was not to copy anyone else's movement, but rather to sense and feel for oneself what is the best and the most efficient way to execute a movement using only your own sensation, experience, and understanding to guide you (Feldenkrais, 1972). The emphasis and focus was that observing your own sensations and feelings while executing a movement has more value than trying to perform what you consider to be the 'correct' movement. Dr. Feldenkrais felt that society places too much value on outside images and not enough on internal esthetics and the sensing of one's Self. He observed that people generally search outside of themselves for models of what they should think—or what they 'should feel' or what they 'should look like'—when deciding whether a movement is 'correct.' When a person is guided by verbal directions to discover what is 'correct' for themselves through their own sensations, the use of an external image is not useful.

However, external images are the most important aspect required to be able to see precisely and clearly what you are looking at in a typically developing child (Stern, 1985; Gage et al., 2009; Konner, 2010). Only in this way is it possible to clearly see what an atypically developing child is doing while in motion. It has much less to do with people finding what is best or more efficient for themselves.

1.3   Observe, describe, do, apply

With this in mind, Dr. Feldenkrais's model of self-learning could no longer be used, because the visual image itself was the crucial starting point and primary building block of my work, i.e., learning how to see a child in motion. This requires the observer

- to use external visual images;
- to understand these images;
- to recognize clearly all the details of movement within the image; and, subsequently,
- to convert them into specific movements related to early development.

Videos of typically developing children—even videos lasting only 15 seconds—contain too much visual information, whereas static photos are completely void of any movement. A good starting point seemed to be a series of photos of infants and young babies in clear sequential moments of movement. I have four children. Watching their early developmental stages of movement held me in rapt fascination, and I spent hundreds of hours documenting each child in videos and photos. It never occurred to me how valuable this enormous trove of photos would become for my later work.

Observe: The first step was to print these photos on large poster boards. This generated many developmental sequences of movements. It was then possible to design and produce many very clear sequences of movement from these thousands of photos of children in motion (Figure 1.1).

The next undertaking was to bring these static images to life, to create an 'image in motion.' The large sequences needed to be broken down into singular elements of just one movement (Figure 1.2). In this format, there is only one frame and one static element to look at. Observing a static photo gives time to look for details in that which is seen without movement. Taking the next static photo in the sequence and going back and forth between the two static photos on a large screen creates a singular movement occurring between the two static images, i.e., one element of movement taking place between two static images. To see the images and to see the change means seeing the singular element of motion itself.

There are an enormous number of categories of children's movements while they are in motion. Putting these categorical observations into words gives others useful ways to practice their own powers of observation to enable them to make discoveries for themselves (Feynman, 1999; Çelik Alexander, 2017). The way to implement this is to pose questions while looking at just one photograph and give categories of specific aspects to observe, as well as a manner in which to observe them. This helps to inhibit one's usual way of looking and focus on the detail in the movement that needs to be discovered at a specific time.

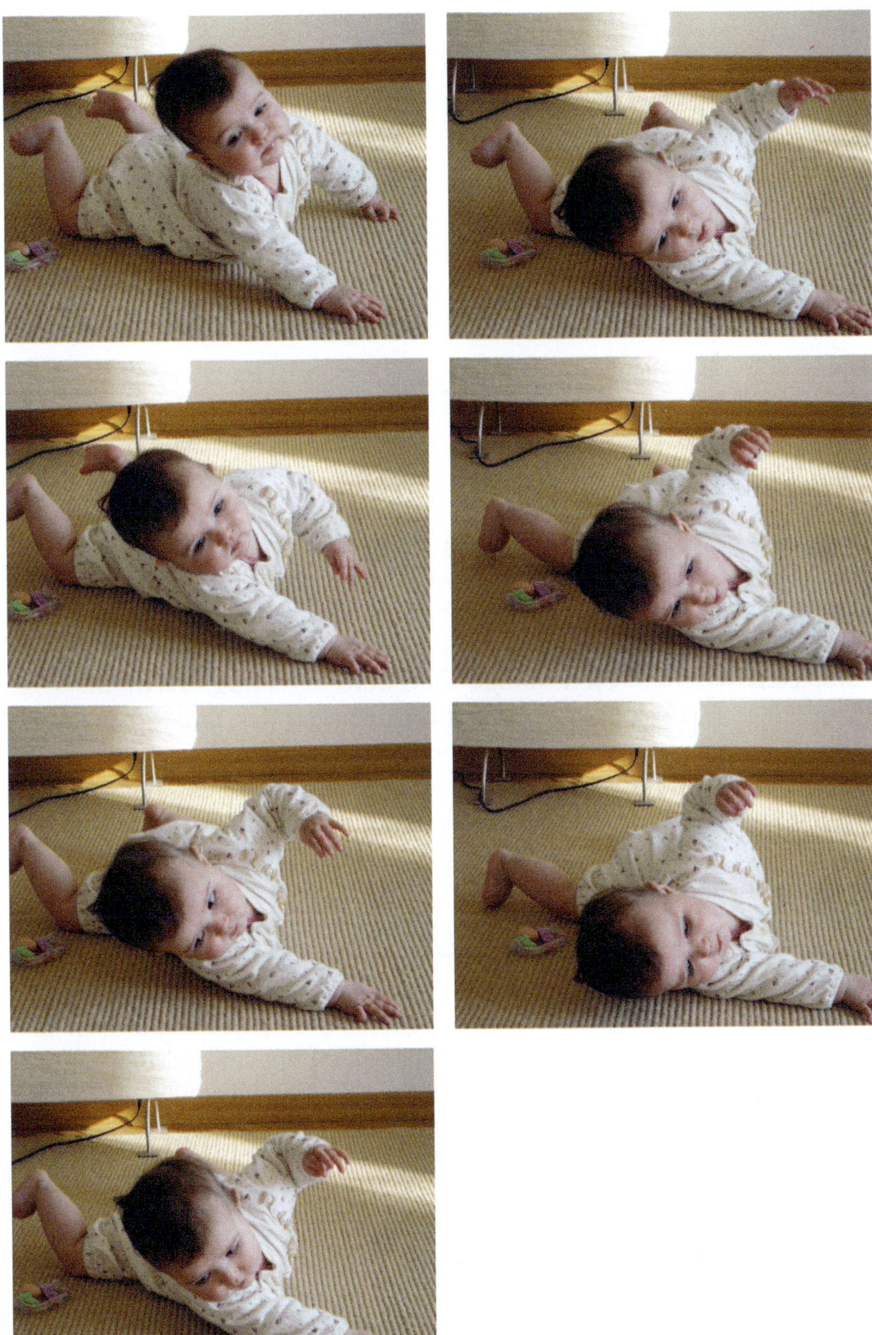

Figure 1.1: Observe and describe

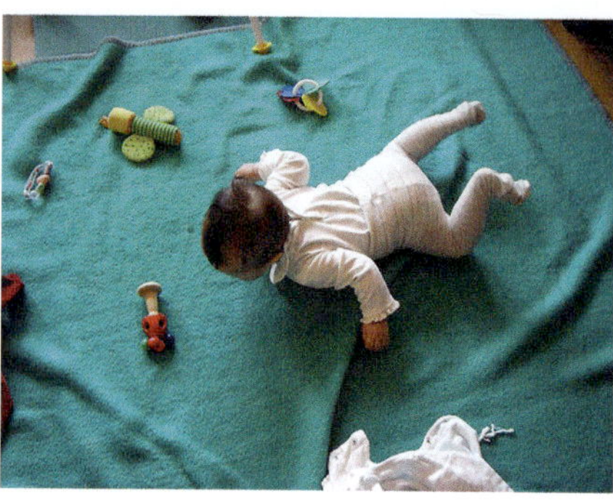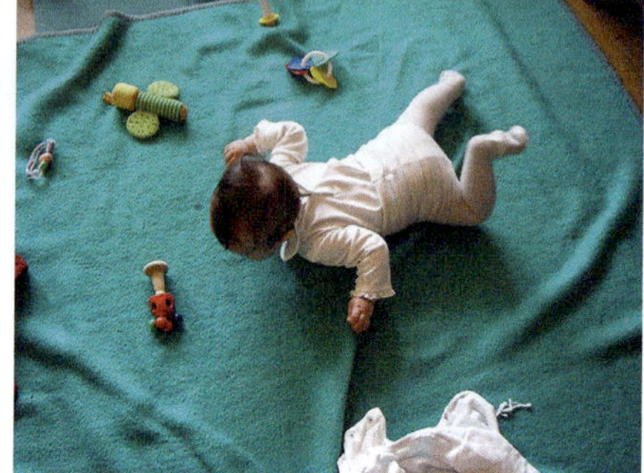

Figure 1.2: Compare movement sequences

In this way, the heuristic and self-discovery method of learning is respected, while transferring and applying it to a very new and different approach.

Describe: I was excited to try out this new approach. The results of presenting this 'observational project' initially came as a great surprise: although the parameters within which to make the observations were provided, the descriptions that came back from the participants were all completely different, even though they were observing exactly the same thing (Hanson, 1958; Siegel, 2007). It became clear that rather than vocally reporting observations, it would be better to have others write them down and make descriptions on paper. It seemed important to concretize the observations. This proved tedious for many, but the labor was not in vain, as it allowed two key elemental foundations to be put into place: *observation and description* (Feynman, 1999).

In the movement sequence shown in Figure 1.1, there is no numbering. When you first look at the photos, do you think there is an order? If so, is it from top to bottom or from bottom to top, or, alternatively, from left to right? Pay attention to what automatically draws your attention.

The order of the photos in the sequence is from top to bottom, starting on the left side and continuing to the top right. There are many elements to observe in this sequence. The first is the overall motion of the head. The head follows a continuous pendular arch-like movement, starting from a more vertical position and ending with the side of the head lying on the floor.

The head moves in relation to the pelvis, starting mostly over the pelvis and ending with a complete twist relative to the pelvis. The pelvis itself remains relatively unchanged. The view of the pelvis changes during the course of the head movement, until the side of the head lies on the floor.

In each of the seven photos, it can be seen that the child's eyes look in different directions relative to its head, sometimes moving with the head and sometimes separately. The right arm remains straight during the entire sequence. The left arm begins straight, then bends at the elbow, making a continuous movement until the elbow ends up pointing directly at the ceiling. The fingers of the left hand start out straight and then continuously bend until the last photo on the bottom right, while the fingers of the right hand remain unchanged.

Notice that both feet and the lower legs slowly straighten and descend toward the floor at different rates.

At first glance, it may seem that the photos in Figure 1.2 are identical. However, when going back and forth between the two and taking a closer look, there are many differences to notice.

Looking at the legs and feet on the left side, both are bent, off the floor, in different positions and at different angles. In the photo on the right, the right leg is on the floor with the heel turned inwards, and the left leg is bent at the knee, so that the sole of the foot is directed toward the ceiling with the knee raised. The left hip joint area also has a much straighter angle than in the photo on the left.

It can also be seen that the positions of the arms, forearms, hands, and fingers are very different between the two photos. In the photo on the left, the right elbow is closer to the trunk than in the right photo. In the photo on the left, the bend in the left elbow has a more open angle than in the photo on the right, in which the elbow is more closed. Also, the directions of the forearms, hands, and fingers are turned in different directions relative to the floor. In the photo on the right, the forearm, thumb, and index fingers are directed more toward the ceiling, whereas in the photo on the left, they are directed more toward the floor.

Do: The next step would be to have the students actually do the movement they had observed and described. The crucial part was that they would need to perform the movement exactly according to their written description. If the description was accurate, the movement would be too. This now completed a three-pronged process of self-discovery:

- observation (visual),
- description (verbal, in written form), and
- doing (movement).

If my reasoning was correct, then the students should now have accomplished the goal: to clearly see what there is to be seen when looking at a child in motion, achieved through a process of self-discovery and embedded in a sensorimotor experience. However, the results of the first attempt were not as I had imagined: when the students actually did the movement they had observed and described, all their movements were different. Again, it was as if they had all seen and described different photos.

After having clarified the first three key elements, the final element to include would be to learn how to implement specific practical therapeutic applications from the particulars of what had been observed, described, and done. An exciting pedagogical tool was now available to put into action.

Apply: Slowly, the realization dawned that these failed attempts had actually succeeded in bringing the entire point of my work into focus. The students were not seeing clearly what they were looking at in a child in motion. To see clearly, you must see what is actually there to be seen, and not what you think is there. If you are looking at a child in motion and seeing, with your perceptual skills, something that differs from that which the child is actually doing, then you will perceptualize your approach: you bring your own perception of what you think the child is doing, and thereupon assess and decide what to do with the child based on your false perception. You will then come and touch the child with this idea 'in your hands.' Thus, you are not seeing or touching this particular child and what this child is doing or needs, but rather you are acting on your own idea of what you think the child is doing. With this false idea, you do not 'meet' the child and its movements or specific needs; you meet your own ideas, perceptions, and movements. This creates a mismatch of sensation, movement, and perception. Once this is understood practically and experientially, the critical importance of having the skill and clarity to observe, describe, and do for working with special needs children becomes apparent.

1.4 Concentrated focusing of attention

When learning how to see what you are looking at in a child in motion through observing, describing, and doing, it is vital to know how and where to focus your attention. One of the first steps toward an unbiased perspective is to recognize that we all have personal tendencies regarding the use of our attention, and we concentrate automatically on what stands out and draws our interest and attention. This becomes very evident while learning this skill set.

Understanding why we are attracted to see one thing and not another is not as important as knowing that this happens automatically, which allows us to be cognizant of when it happens (Thelen & Smith, 1994; Bainbridge-Cohen, 1994). Learning to use the skill of focusing is important, as it lets us filter out what is not important in a particular moment in order to concentrate and see that which is essential. This is of great importance when working with a special needs child.

The skill of focusing is learned gradually in a variety of ways. The basic aspects are

- focusing,
- focusing on single elements,
- focusing on combinations of elements, and
- focusing on patterns.

Initially, one needs to be able to focus in general. This means intentionally and voluntarily taking charge of one's ability to focus and directing it toward something in a purposeful manner. To do this, you need to learn how to inhibit the tendency to be drawn toward whatever is demanding and attracts your attention at the onset.

Focusing on single elements: Once this is clear, it is possible to learn how to focus on single elements. For this, static photos of babies in motion are first introduced, followed by video. Tasks of singling out very specific parts of a child's movement are set to develop this skill.

Focusing on combinations of elements: After practicing this many times, identifying just one element from a large number of competing components of a movement and skillfully focusing on this single element begins to become easier. Once this skill set is learned, it is possible to start learning how to focus on combinations. This requires learning to see the way in which two or more elements of a child's movement interact and combine with each other in various ways; some combinations are similar to one another, others are different. Learning how to focus on combinations confers the skill to observe the same or similar elements combining in movement in a variety of ways in different situations, as well as in different relations to gravity.

These skills allow you to begin to focus on a child in motion and pick out only the specific elements of the entire movement that you want to or need to focus on. This is a very important stage, as it represents an opportunity to clearly point out that which needs to be observed. It provides the opportunity to recognize, clearly see, and follow the movement, and to identify any changes that may take place in the distinct elements that are in focus.

Focusing on patterns: The next facet of learning this skill set is to be able to focus on patterns. To focus on a pattern of movement is to learn how to clearly discern the ways in which single elements and combinations of elements combine to form a pattern of movement or movement behavior. A pattern is something that repeats itself on a regular basis (Feynman, 1999; Bainbridge-Cohen, 1994; Thelen & Smith, 1993; Edelman, 2006). There are many kinds of patterns in many domains. Patterns of language and speech are good, easy-to-understand examples. Another commonly understood pattern type is a weather pattern. In this work, the focus is on how to observe patterns of movement. To see the regularity and repetition, and clearly recognize how a pattern repeats itself, is a necessary skill when working in the domain of therapeutic learning focused on movement. When something is moving slowly, and the repetition is identical each time, it is easier to focus in on the details of how all the single elements and combinations of elements combine to form the pattern. However, when the pattern does not repeat itself in exactly the same way every time, and the rhythms of the movement vary—sometimes slowly, sometimes quickly, and sometimes a bit of both—it is not so easy to focus in on and clearly recognize a pattern.

Each of these four components of focusing are essential skills required to clearly observe movement in both children and adults, as well as when working in almost all domains that deal with movement for therapeutic and learning purposes. Focusing is a crucial skill for working effectively with special needs children. Focusing is studied by first learning each of the separate components with typically developing children and then transferring and applying these skills to atypically developing children. Having good focusing skills allows for much more efficient and distinct ways of identifying what a child needs during the time you have working together. They enable you to assess clearly if and when the child shows improvement and progress. These skills also lend greater competence when explaining to others what you are looking at, why you are doing what you are doing, and how to see the changes in the movement of the child.

No two children are alike in terms of the individual ways in which they move. This is particularly true of special needs children with the challenges they face while in motion. Given these challenges, there is a much wider variety of possible movement combinations, configurations, and patterns to know and be skillful in focusing upon.

I depend upon this concentrated kind of focusing daily in my private practice. A child often arrives in my office with one or both parents, perhaps a grandmother or a nanny, and very often a sibling or even two. The child may be excited or anxious or both. The sibling wants to play, the parents want to ask questions and tell me things, and the child I will work with is moving constantly in chaotic ways or in a certain rhythm, making sounds, or talking, depending upon the condition they present. In such a situation it is important to be able to let the surrounding stimuli and conversation continue while focusing in on the child with whom you will work. You must be able to focus directly and specifically on the essential aspects of the child's movement and behavior. Your assessment of what you need to do, how you should act, the voice you should use with the child, and where to begin must be clear and precise. You must also focus your attention on the child to reassure them of a safe environment. This can all be happening while the parents are asking questions, the sibling may be running around and grabbing toys, and the grandmother is telling the child to sit quietly.

Abilities orientation 2

As adults, we need to keep in mind that we can never really comprehend the movements of a baby, as our skeleton, our muscles, and our brain are already further developed. We need to be aware of our own preconceived ideas, expectations, and evaluations when watching a child. An ability-oriented approach is not focused on impairments and deficiencies but rather concentrates on potentials.[1] Recognizing these potentials and empathically communicating them in the therapeutic relationship and learning situation can promote the emergence, development, and stabilization of abilities.

2.1 Abilities rather than disabilities

We all have some kind of perspective on movement, learning, therapy, and exercise. It is important to dwell for a moment on the perspective we have on the early development of movement in relation to both typically and atypically developing children.

Viewpoints and frames of reference: When we think of, observe, or watch a typically developing child during the first two years of life, as it is developing its movement repertoire from lying on its back all the way up to walking, talking, hopping, and jumping, everyone imagines a healthy, robust, active baby developing more and more abilities, skills, and competencies in moving around in space, exploring new parts of itself and its surroundings, and in relating to others. We focus primarily on the typically developing child's *abilities*.

DOI: 10.4324/9781003737988-2

When we shift our focus to observing motion and behavior in an atypically developing child, most of us will have a very strong tendency—if not a completely overriding compulsion—to look at the child's *disabilities*: what they *cannot do*, what they have *never done*, ways in which they *do not move*, how they have *not reached* yet another milestone of movement development, etc. The negative becomes the prime emphasis and perspective. The way of observing the child, relating to the child, sensing, and feeling the child all adopt the viewpoint of the *disability*, the lack of skill, the lack of a means to accomplish, the lack of a competence. This in itself creates a vision of the child who is unable and lacking. It forwards a thinking that the child must be fixed, corrected, made 'normal.' From the perspective of a therapist or parent, this has many ramifications in the personal and practical domains.

Self-identity and relationships: A child comes to sense, feel, understand itself, and form their personal identity through how we relate to them. When we relate to a child in words, in touch, and via nonverbal communication in terms of what they cannot do, this is also how the child comes to know themselves as a person. The child's identity and self-image are formed by how we interact with and deal with them (Heller & LaPierre, 2012; Schore, 1994). This is true not only in the familial and social domains, but takes on even stronger relevance in a therapeutic learning situation. Not only how we look at and relate to the child's challenges, but also how we touch the child in any kind of therapeutic manner is important. If the focus of the therapist's hands is to 'get rid of the problem,' this is what the therapist will find—problems, difficulties, and disability. If the focus is to try to make the child do something they cannot, the child senses and feels that they cannot; the nervous system will respond to this in such a way that the child cannot. If the therapist's hands seek the child's abilities—no matter how difficult the objective challenges of the child may seem—they will find them, and the nervous system will respond accordingly.

This is not to say that an atypically developing child does not face objective challenges or require assistance in a variety of spheres on the path to more independence.

Abilities and potentials: Speaking of abilities rather than disabilities is not a matter of semantics, but rather a very practical issue for those who are related to and work with special needs children.

Not all atypically developing children are born with special needs. There are children who develop atypically from birth, and there are children who develop typically for a time and then, later on, due to certain reasons and circumstances, become children with special needs.

CASE EXAMPLE LINDA—SEEING ABILITIES AND NOT DISABILITIES

Linda is such a child. Until she was 8 years old, Linda developed as a typical, very happy, and socially active child. She loved school, her activities, and her friends. At age 8, her parents started to observe certain difficulties in her coordination every so often. Sometimes things would slip out of her hands, she would miss a step, or a sentence would not come out correctly. The difficulties became much more apparent over time, and not only to her parents. It became clear that there was something affecting Linda, and her parents decided to seek advice. It was sadly discovered that Linda had a brain tumor, which was successfully removed through surgery.

The surgery left Linda with a number of challenges and movement difficulties, particularly balance problems. She had difficulty maintaining balance while sitting and walking and also with walking in straight lines. At Linda's first visit, she could not take more than one step without losing her balance. As the sessions progressed, she learned to walk for much longer periods. Although her ability to walk improved, she was not fully stable on her legs and would often shake and tremble as she walked. Linda was very determined to walk again. She loved her school and friends: her goal was to return to school and be able to walk down the hall with her friends unaided.

During this same period, I was working with a very well-known dancer. Her sessions followed immediately after Linda's. At the time I had a very large room in my private practice that I used for group work. Upon entering the practice, you would go directly into that large space. The rooms where I held private sessions were down a hallway. One day, my session with Linda went on a bit longer, and she wanted to walk in the larger room for a while after her session. The well-known dancer was in that room, walking around and waiting for her session. When Linda walked into the space, the dancer stopped and began watching her attentively. Later, during her session, the dancer told me how taken she was with this young girl, her extraordinary ability 'in the way' she walked, and how elegantly she managed herself, her balance, and her steps. She described Linda as graceful, attentive, and present to herself. She told me she wished that many of her dancers would be as attentive and present as this girl and possess the kind of inner aesthetic that Linda exhibited. I was struck by how this accomplished dancer looked at and perceived only Linda's abilities.

This was a very clear demonstration and statement of the possibility of an ability and not a disability!

When faced with challenges, human nature leads us to seek within to find qualities that we would not normally use or need. This was true of Linda. Her trembling and unstable walking became her gateway to abilities within herself that she would not have needed to focus on had it not been for her surgery and subsequent special needs. Week after week, the dancer would come early to watch Linda walking. At first, Linda did not know who she was. As time went by, they came to know each other. The dancer told her how extraordinary she was and how her walking inspired her and her choreography. There were many moments of pride, success, fear of the unknown, and figuring out during Linda's sessions, and she did reach her goal: she was able to go back to school and walk unaided down the hallway with her friends. I wish I could have been there to see her, but I will never forget the look in her eyes and the expression on her face when she told me about her first day back at school.

Recognize potential: The perspective that I use is one of ability and potential. The focus is first and foremost on what the child can do. The moment you begin to look at any atypically developing child from this standpoint of abilities and potential, you begin to look at a completely different child from the one seen by someone looking from the perspective of disability. Looking from the standpoint of abilities permits perspectives of possibility, change, learning, development, and growth in all domains. This viewpoint translates into very powerful and practical therapeutic learning applications that achieve astonishing results and outcomes.

Develop potential: When an adult relates to a child as an able being who needs assistance to develop their potential, the child senses it. The child senses a person who is looking at them for who they are, and not who they could be without a disability. The child is a whole, just as any other child is, with a brain, muscles, bones, emotions, and sensations. What we find is what we focus on.

See abilities: When a child is touched by a therapist who listens with their hands for where a child can move and what they can do, the child senses this. When the therapist relates to the child as *being able* to do something and maintains this perspective in their manner of working, the results are completely different.

Develop abilities: Focusing on abilities allows you to focus on the uniqueness of the child you are with and their specific way of moving. It makes *room for abilities to develop through movement* and personal engagement with the child. It is an opportunity for the child to gain possession of the means to learn and accomplish something new in a developmental direction. It allows for an outlook of progress and the formation of new abilities and skills.

2.2   Emergence, development, and stabilization of abilities

Progress and growth of an ability and the learning involved often do not follow an even path. Sometimes, during any one of the three stages of ability development, the change is seen to happen very rapidly, and the rate of expansion of the ability is fast. Sometimes we witness a sudden and immediate unexpected change. Other times, the change can be very slow and gradual. There may also be regression in the development, or one ability might seem to grow at a fast rate while another lags behind or doesn't develop at all. Emergence, development, and stability can occur in a variety of spurts and, thus, periods occur during which several abilities, movement patterns, positions, and ways of transitioning intermingle. These phases of spurts and intermingling frequently trigger the emergence of one or more new abilities.

Abilities develop and find form in a typically developing child progressively. There are three basic stages:

1. emergence of an ability,
2. development of an ability, and
3. stabilization of an ability.

The three domains are fluid and may overlap with different abilities.

Emergence: We first see the emergence of an ability. This is like the first new bud of a leaf on a tree in springtime, just as it begins to show itself. It is starting to emerge. Depending on the size of the leaf and the weather, the bud will slowly but surely reveal itself over a period of time. A good example of this in the development of movement is the emergence of rolling from the back to the side to the stomach. We don't see children who learn to roll from one day to the next. What we do see is that the child begins to make certain small movements that start to shift it from being on the back toward being on the side. At the onset, the child doesn't roll completely onto their side, but it is clear that they are moving from their back in the direction of their side. This is what we can call the emergence of the ability to roll from the back onto the side.

Development: After the emergence of an ability, we see its development. This is when the ability that has emerged takes on all its characteristics and makes connections to and adapts other abilities in the child's movement and behavior repertoire. Continuing with the example of rolling, we observe that in the developmental phase of the ability to roll, a child will explore, try out, and become successful in rolling from their back to their side and returning to their back, and in rolling from their back to their side and then onto their stomach, and also from starting on their side and rolling onto their stomach. A child will do this with their head sometimes off and sometimes on the ground; starting sometimes from their feet or legs, sometimes from their hands or arms, and sometimes from their eyes and head. As the development of the ability progresses, the child will develop a large variety of ways to roll.

Stabilization: Finally, we see the stabilization of the ability. This means that the ability has developed to such a degree that it is a clear ability which the child uses more and more in their daily life. Sticking with rolling, we will see the child roll from their back to their stomach and return to their back with their raised head off of the ground the entire time. This does not, however, imply that once the ability is stable in the early situations of back, side, and stomach, that the *ability to roll* will not continue to grow and improve. All abilities can constantly improve. The ability to roll (Figure 2.1) continues to develop further into rolling from all sorts of positions, higher in gravity.

Looking at abilities from the viewpoint of the emergence, development, and stability of an ability is a helpful tool to observe and assess any ability that a child is developing (Schore, 1994; Fogel, 2013). When observing special needs children, it is especially useful, as it provides a means for deciphering which abilities are at the emergent stage, which are at the developing stage, and which abilities of the child are in a stable stage. Children developing with special needs often present a large mixture of abilities in the emergent, developing, and stable stages. With these children in particular, it is often seen that some abilities do not pass through from one stage to another. This, in turn, may have an effect on the emergence, development, or stability of another ability. Learning to see this intermingling of the different stages is a first step toward finding a way to intervene and let growth and progress in the abilities continue in a positive and efficient way.

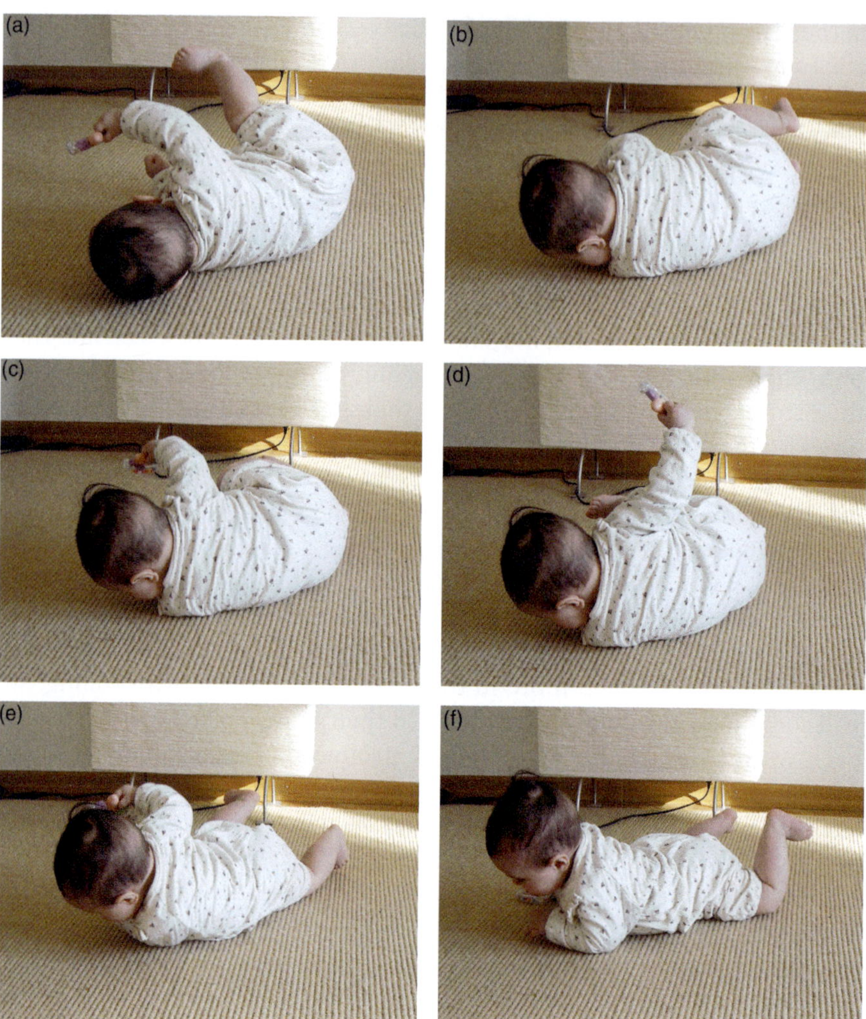

Figure 2.1: Rolling from the back onto the stomach

The movement sequence in Figure 2.1 complements a movement exploration found in the 'try it for yourself' rolling movement exploration below. The sequence shown in the photos is just one of many ways in which a child rolls onto their stomach. It is an example of how the head and eyes guide and organize movements of the body. In this sequence, once the child's head is lifted into the air and turned toward the floor, it remains lifted, creating a side-bending and maintaining tone that allows the child to roll onto their stomach.

In photo a), the head is on the side. The shoulder and pelvis, elbow and knee, and foot and hand are aligned with each other.

In photo b), the head turns so that the face and eyes are directed toward the floor. The head and eyes will now remain in this direction throughout the entire sequence, while the rest of the body now organizes itself to turn relative to the head and come onto the stomach. The shoulder and the pelvis remain in the same line, but the elbow and knee and the foot and the hand do not. There is a shortening of the right side of the body and a lengthening of the left.

In photo c), the head lifts slightly more away from the floor while the right knee and thigh come a bit lower to the floor. The right hand and elbow bend slightly and lift away from the floor, yet the line between the pelvis and the shoulder remains unchanged. Movement in the shoulder and hip joints is necessary for this to take place.

In photo d), the right leg extends forward, accompanied by the right side of the pelvis. This happens at the same time as the right arm and right shoulder continue to go backward.

In photo e), the right leg moves down to the floor and in the direction of the feet, creating more extension in the back and allowing the upper body to roll over the left shoulder. This begins to pull and bring the right arm forward, creating momentum. The left leg can now be seen to straighten downward.

In photo f) the child arrives on their stomach with their head lifted, back extended, and left forearm and elbow on the floor.

The development of rolling onto the side and the stomach with the head lifted and maintained in the air the entire time is an important ability to develop.

Movement—a complex ability: As an adult it is difficult to appreciate the complexity of these stages because the early developing patterns of movement and abilities are stable and fully formed. As adults, we cannot undo our knowledge of 'how to do' something. To appreciate the developing child in motion, we must first appreciate that they have never done it before and, thus, have no previous experience to rely on, and that their motivation to roll or execute any new movement is different. It is possible, however, to try rolling for yourself, to demonstrate experimentally that rolling is a complex ability.

Try it yourself—rolling

- Find a comfortable space on the floor and lie down on your back.
- Imagine not knowing how to roll and try to move in such a way that you only execute the beginnings of a roll onto your side and return to your back. After this, try to roll completely onto your side and return to your back.

- The next step would be to roll from your back onto your stomach and back again, with your head in the air all the time, while not pushing with either your arms, elbows, feet, or knees. If you pay close attention, you will find that there are many details to coordinate.
- Now take another moment to try out a few different ways to roll.
- From what position do you begin? Where do you end up? Do you do it easily? Smoothly? Is it bumpy or awkward? If you had to explain the movement in words to someone who cannot roll, could you? In how many ways can you roll? What different kinds of rolls have you mastered?

2.3   Baby movements and adult movements

To learn how to experience developmental ideas through movement and apply this knowledge to work with special needs children and/or adults, it is of prime importance to understand that adults cannot perform 'baby movements.'

When looking at a baby's skeleton, musculature, and brain, it becomes very clear that they are different from those of an adult in all respects. We really cannot do 'baby movements.' The postnatal infant has no set structure and is very amenable to change during the early growth phases; thus, it has no preset development of function. The structure and function of these three systems—skeleton, musculature, and brain—continue to expand and evolve through their interaction with gravity and the social and physical environment. These interactions and experiences also have an impact on gene expression.

Early on in my teaching of the development of movement, I discovered that there is a gross misconception and misunderstanding of this idea. Many workshop participants, professionals, and parents think that when early developmental movement is studied in an experiential way, that the movements performed are 'baby movements.'

I noticed that many people try to infer what a baby is feeling, sensing, and thinking, and try to put themselves in a baby-like state when executing the movements: they try to feel like babies, and they try to act like babies while they are moving. People seem to think that this gives them a clearer understanding of the movement being performed, felt, and sensed by the baby. They try to 'regress' into what they think is an earlier emotional and sensorimotor state of being. However, this leads to great confusion, because an adult cannot perform 'baby movements.' An adult also cannot sense or feel 'baby sensations' or 'baby feelings,' or experience 'baby thinking.'

The confusion is further exacerbated when this kind of thinking is transferred to working with a child in a therapeutic learning situation. An adult simply cannot be a baby in any domain—most certainly not in the domain of movement—and this approach leads to tremendous misunderstanding, particularly when applied to a special needs child. Although this may seem obvious to some, many people disagree with me on this point. But is it not crystal clear that a baby is not an adult in any domain? A baby has a different skeleton, different musculature, a different brain, and a different set of emotions, sensations, and cognitive abilities within a different framework than does an adult. Let us take a moment and look at a few of these aspects.

Development of the skeleton, muscles, and brain: To begin with, all of a baby's systems are developing systems, not developed systems, as in an adult.

A baby's skeleton is a forming, undeveloped skeleton. Its proportions are completely different from those of an adult skeleton.

The joints in the spine of an infant are not formed in the same way as those in an adult skeleton. The human skeleton starts to form in the very early days of pregnancy in utero and continues to develop and grow until a person is between 20 and 25 years of age. Bones grow rapidly during childhood and throughout puberty. The development and growth of all bones of the human skeleton is a complex process entailing much more than just getting longer and larger. An adult spine has three major curves, and it takes over 20 years for them to fully form.

It is also important to point out that these three major curves are not present in the young baby and only develop through the variety of movements that a baby performs in the different positions they learn while moving during the first years of life.

The musculature of a baby is very different to that of an adult. Like the skeleton, human musculature forms and begins to develop in utero, and undergoes tremendous changes once the baby is born and gravity begins to play a role. The muscle fibers of a young baby continuously grow and increase in size.

During the first year of life, the baby slowly develops more and more strength as well as the coordination and skill necessary to accomplish intentional and purposeful movements and activities. The baby does not yet think in words and cannot yet self-regulate for the most part in almost any domain. The baby goes through a gradual process of gaining control of and using their musculature in a variety of situations and positions in gravity. They gain strength and control over their arms, legs, head, and chest, and they gradually become able to accomplish more and more movements and activities higher and higher up in gravity.

At birth, a baby's brain is not fully developed. It doubles in size during the first year of life and continues to grow rapidly for the first five years until it reaches 90% of the size of the future adult brain. A very important function of a baby's brain is the continuous formation of new neural connections and establishment of neural networks through continuous interaction, stimulation, experience, and movement. The interactions and movements in a baby are both active and reactive, and these actions and reactions contribute to formation of these neural connections and networks. A nurturing, supportive, and safe environment that encourages communication and play helps in the process of healthy brain development in a child. An adult's neural networks are fully formed. Adults can still engage in learning and modify these networks, but certainly not in the same way or at the same rate as a baby's brain can.

The same is true for *emotions and perceptions*. These are learned and develop during the first years of life through interaction with the primary care giver(s) and others, through movement, contact, and through touch. Adults have emotional reactions and feelings which have meanings related to the perceptions which make up their realities.

Along the path to development of structure and function, emotional and perceptual interpretations of reality become intertwined to create a child's *functional, social, perceptual,* and *emotional identities*. As adults, these identities are already formed.

As a baby is developing, growing, and using large varieties of movements, their neuromusculoskeletal system and brain grow and learn how to adapt to complex situations in behavior. The baby needs to become an independent walker and talker. If given a rich, safe, and stimulating environment, the baby will develop in all aspects necessary to become an independent person. A baby uses what they have and what is present in their social and physical environment to constantly improve in all ways. As the baby grows and learns, they adapt to all kinds of situations and slowly develop habits that suit their needs in coping and adjusting to these situations. An adult has a formed structure, habits of function, and set ways of perceiving, sensing, and acting.

Movement possibilities in adults: To improve movement as an adult and to learn how to function in an easier and more efficient way, we must first 'deconstruct' our movements into smaller elements and patterns. Part of this learning comprises how to use our attention during movement to discover the set habits and self-imposed limitations we have conferred to our movements in our own personal ways. Once we begin to do this, we open ourselves once more to fundamental qualities of change and learning, so that our skeletal, muscular, and nervous systems can begin to have new sensorimotor experiences. We perform 'adult movements' which permit change and growth.

The three curves of the spine can be used as an example to illustrate this point. The movements of a baby in various positions in gravity provide the stimuli to the neuromusculoskeletal system necessary to develop a curve. The baby's curves are flexible in all directions, and its skeleton can combine the three developing curves in an assortment of ways, as determined by the baby's movements.

An adult's three curves are fully formed. If we want to appreciate from the perspective of an adult what it feels like to develop the curves of our spine, we can attempt to imitate different kinds of movements of the baby during the formation of the curves. However, this is only an approximation of what the baby actually does, as we cannot change the curves of a formed adult structure. The structural curves of the spine can become more flexible, but they cannot behave in the same way as a baby's curves, which are actually formed by such movements during early childhood development.

This is why we cannot do 'baby movements' or more precisely 'early formative movements.' What we can do as adults is to 'deconstruct' our adult movements, but these deconstructions are not 'baby movements.'

Try it yourself—baby movements

Movement exploration:

- Take a moment to lie on your back with your legs fully extended. Notice that many parts of your spine do not contact the floor and that you have three spinal curves.
- Try for a moment to completely flatten the curves. First, try to flatten each one separately and then all three together. If you really try hard, you will be forced into all sorts of contortions in an effort to succeed, but you will not be successful. Even if you feel you are able to do it to some degree, it should become very clear that it is not your bones that change and flatten, but that you are simply pressing one area harder into the floor for a moment.

Movement experiment:

- Another example to try with the curves of the spine is to lie on the floor with your legs extended or bent, and try to flatten just the curve of your neck (Figure 2.2)

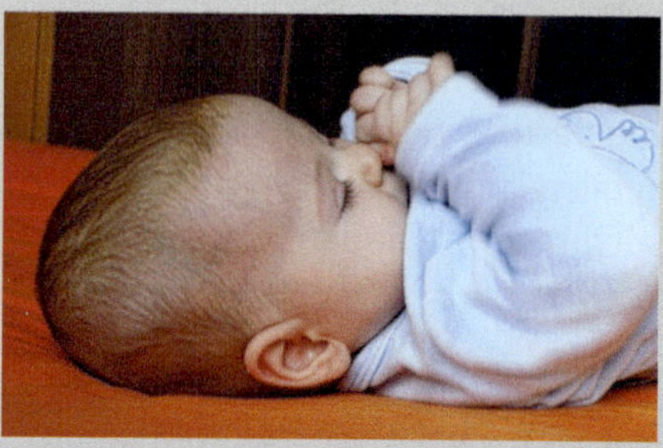

Figure 2.2:
Modifying the curves of the spine

- Most of us will become attentive and aware, and observe that we lift some other part of our spine when trying to do this. The baby does not need to lift their spine.
- If you try to bring your lower back fully down to the floor, you will most likely tighten your belly muscles and/or lift your chest.
- If you now simultaneously try to flatten all three curves of your spine, you will most likely find yourself straining, contorting, and holding your breath. It will feel unnatural.
- As soon as you stop trying to flatten your lower back, it will leave the floor again. For a baby, flattening their spine is a normal everyday movement.

If we, as adults, execute movements while attending in various ways to what we do and how we do it, we can discover habits we have unwittingly developed in our movements and readily improve our overall abilities and way of moving. I will discuss this in more detail later, in the section entitled 'JKA—Abilities Lessons in Movement' (see Chapter 10.2).

Note

1. The term 'potentials' and 'potential development' are oriented toward the ideas of Gerald Hüther (Hüther, 2023).

Primary elements of movements **3**

Planning, control, tone, and balance are the primary components of any movement. If these cooperate appropriately, the effect is flowing, light, purposeful, and efficient. To enable coordination, integration, and networking of these four components, a complex interplay between nerves, the musculoskeletal system, and mental, emotional, and social factors is required. Experiential learning aims to enable a differentiated perception of the quality of movements or elements thereof, and of the interplay between sensation, movement, and action.

3.1 Kinesthetic clarity

In many cases it is not only the movement itself that a child needs in order to foster change, but also the understanding of how to apply a particular movement to a particular primary component. Clarity of sensation (kinesthetic clarity) is an essential movement experience. It is another important cornerstone of experiential learning, which makes it possible to work effectively with special needs children. In order to create and facilitate emergence and development of change in a child, it is necessary to appreciate the child's experiential world in the sensation–movement–action domain.

One first needs to grasp these qualities and subtleties within oneself and have very distinct sensory experiences within one's own body and movements (Fogel, 2013; Feldenkrais, 1981; Rywerant, 1983). These qualities and subtleties need to be sensed and elucidated in personal experience; they must not exist exclusively in the cognitive domain.

DOI: 10.4324/9781003737988-3

Kinesthetic perception: Frequently, when a special needs child experiences something new in movement, it is accompanied by a specific sensation. The child needs to be able to distinguish, feel, and identify this separately from the myriad of other sensations they are constantly engaged with. The child may be very young, nonverbal, or have challenges in the sensori-motor, emotional, or cognitive domain. Yet something new appearing for the child can easily be seen with trained eyes and felt with skilled hands. New, unmistakable sensations which appear during the learning process need to be respected, valued, and encouraged during the moments of the experience itself.

An adult attempting to help the child in this way must come to appreciate the specificity and effects of these sensory encounters. This is only possible after experiencing first-hand contact with the effects of what I have come to call *back-and-forth movements* and the impressions that these movements have on us.

Back-and-forth movements: The discovery of back-and-forth movements was a revelation. I found that executing the same movement back and forth a short number of times produces a very specific sensation. These sensations are clear and kinesthetically distinguishable. They are generated by executing a singular movement in a back-and-forth manner. The specific effects that arise are also reproducible. If repeated in the same way on a different day, they will produce the same specific perceivable sensation. Distinguishable, clear, and particular kinesthetic sensations allow us to experience what I have defined as *kinesthetic clarity*. Individual inner impressions such as length, width, roundness, shortness, uprightness, flatness, lightness, and heaviness are a few of these. Regardless of the background one has in movement, personally or professionally, the effects are immediate, perceivable, and similar.

Kinesthetic clarity and movements: Kinesthetic clarity is only achievable with one or possibly two combinations of back-and-forth movements. When the movement sequence is longer, the sensations become more diffuse, making it difficult to make sharp, clear-cut, specific sensory distinctions. There is a certain threshold at which clarity of sensation becomes blurred, and the kinesthetic experience becomes a more generalized movement process experience. This also has value, but of a very different kind. The longer and more complex the movement process becomes, the more sensations, emotions, and perceptions are evoked. If a process goes on for longer than 20 or 30 minutes—involving a wide variety of movements as well as pauses and linked to different kinds of attentional states—there can be no kinesthetic clarity. For an adult, the experience of a long movement sequence can be pleasant and beneficial, and it can evoke an overall change in the individual's sense of musculoskeletal organization. However, the sharpness and clarity that can be discerned in one very specific sensation produced by a specific movement is lost in a long sequence.

The field of kinesthetic comprehension, learning, and experience is not new. Scientists, educators, artists, and architects of the late 19th century took part in many wide-ranging discussions on these topics. The architectural historian Zeynep Çelik Alexander writes about this in her book, *Kinaesthetic Knowing* (Çelik Alexander, 2017). The understanding, experience, and use of 'back-and-forth movements' is a further contribution to this aspect of education.

3.2   Planning, control, tone, and balance

There are four primary components of every voluntary movement: planning, control, tone, and balance. When all four components orchestrate to function together in a smooth and integrated fashion, we experience a well-coordinated action from the inside, and a well-coordinated action can be observed from the outside.

Planning, control, tone, and balance

An understanding of these four primary components—how they interact with and influence one another—guides us in how to evaluate and interact with a child, or how to support the child in

- planning,
- improving possibilities for control,
- raising or lowering tonus,
- the various ways in which to improve balance while moving and maintaining various positions.

Simultaneously, the observer's understanding of these four components

- provides the observer with a good vantage point from which to evaluate and interact with the child's neuromusculoskeletal system, in order to
- facilitate improvement of the physical, mental, sensory, and emotional domains.

The growth of functional abilities is a complex process of networking between different parts of the brain, the musculoskeletal system, and the external social and physical environment. This process of networking, of coordinating, and of integrating among the four primary components of movement leads to more voluntary action and a constant increase in the child's repertoire of movement and action skills. The importance of identifying which aspect of the four primary components needs to develop or improve and how to facilitate this is a key element in the teaching of my approach (Figure 3.1).

Planning: When we are about to execute any type of movement, we must have some kind of internal plan or model of what it is we want to do. There needs to be some form of image of the movement: Which parts of the body will be moving? How will they be moving? Where will they be moving to in relation to one another? How are the different movements of different body parts coordinated with one another? This planning takes place in various parts of the brain and is dependent to a large extent on personal experience (Feldenkrais, 1972; Rywerant, 1983; Edelman, 2006). For example, if you want to grab an orange out of a bowl, you first need to have an interest in the orange. Then, you direct yourself toward it, and because you have tried to reach, grab, and take an orange many times before, the movement is already formed in your experience. Thus, you just reach and grab. Yet, if we think for a moment of how many trials and errors a baby must endure in learning to reach out to grab something which has a certain weight, shape, and color, we can see that there are many fine details involved in successfully completing this movement. We must know how far away the orange is; we must learn to judge the distance between ourself and the orange; we must decide what it is we need to move first—the hand? The fingers? The shoulder blade? The back? We need to know if the orange will fit into one hand or if we need both; how hard do we need to close our hand(s) around the orange, so that it won't fall out? How much strength do we need in our arm to lift the orange and bring it back to us? Grabbing for an orange is actually a very intricate procedure with many variables.

A very young child explores and plays with each and every one of these variables until able to successfully complete the movement. Once it is successful at combining all the elements of such a process, they transfer this schema of the type of planning, reaching, grabbing, and taking something that has a particular weight and store it in their brain as a successfully planned-out action that can be repeated over and over again automatically. The information of this schema is stored not only in terms of one size, color, shape, and weight of 'an orange,' but rather has many variations and forms of this information. Otherwise, for every new kind of 'orange,' we would have to go through the entire process all over again. What we need to remember is that every time we execute the hundreds and thousands of actions we use daily, we have already practiced archetypal models of each type of action hundreds and thousands of times before. To understand this point more clearly, it is easy enough to just observe a child with cerebral palsy who has spastic hands or an adult who has had a stroke, to see how much they need to '(re-)learn' just to reach out and grab an orange!

Control: Once we have a clear idea of what we want to do, the next component that makes up every action is control. We need to be able to control the different parts of our body so that we can accomplish what we have set out to do in an organized manner. We need to be able to put our plan into action and bring it to fruition (Rywerant, 1983; Hüther, 2006; Feldenkrais, 1949). We must be able control the direction, speed, timing, and distances moved by our moving parts while stabilizing our nonmoving parts. We also need to be able to

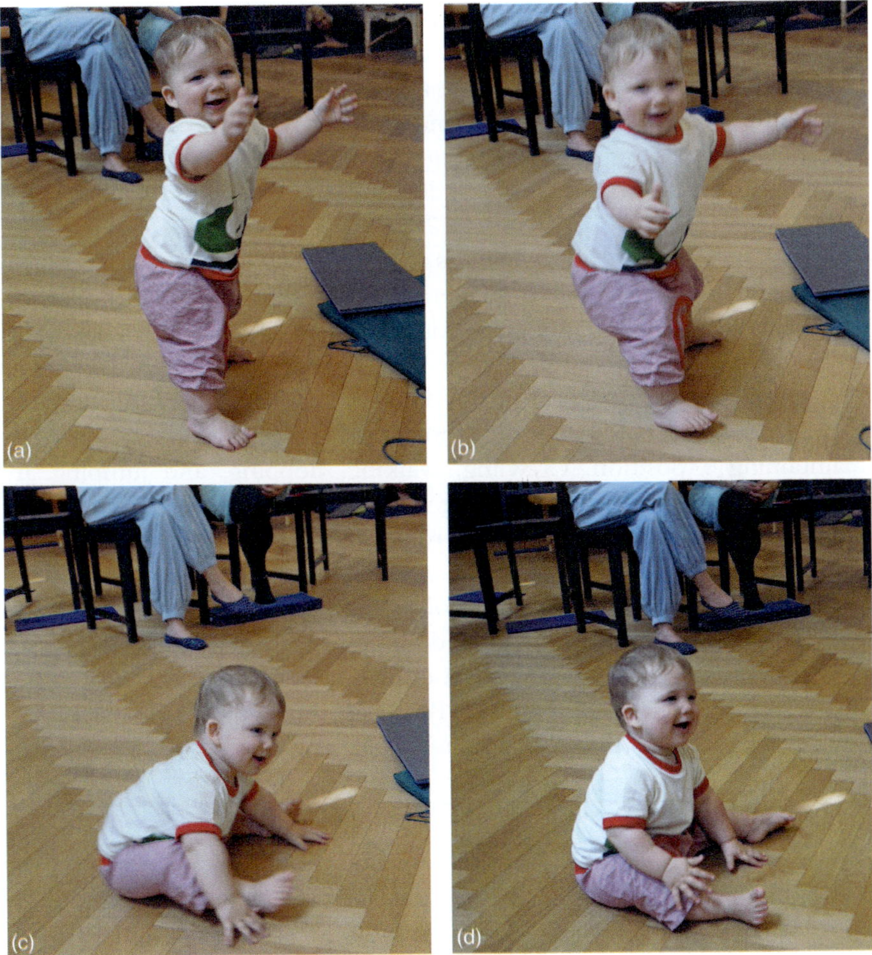

Figure 3.1: Transitioning from standing to sitting

control the strength and force we put into the movement. If any one of these aspects in the control of the movement is not coordinated with other aspects, then the planned intended movement will not be realized and completed.

Tone: While at rest, we have a certain amount of firmness and tautness in our muscles. This firmness can be thought of as the tone or tonus of the muscles. When we begin any movement, we need a degree of firmness. We need to be able to use this tone, this solidity, to begin and end a movement that we want to complete with the appropriate amount of intensity and force. Tone keeps us ready to move and act (Gage et al., 2009; Feldenkrais, 1949). It keeps us from applying excessive force and also keeps us from applying too little force. We need a certain degree of tone to accompany the planning and control of any movement. For any action, we need to muster and precisely use the proper amount of force. If we go back to our 'orange,' the appropriate amount of force allows us to hold it without crushing or dropping it—not too much and not too little. Our tone allows us to move smoothly from one situation in gravity to another and maintain ourselves in upright positions and moving situations, such as rolling up to sitting, moving from sitting to standing, and transitioning from standing to walking.

Balance: Balance can be defined as the ability to maintain and control movements without falling or disrupting the equilibrium. Balance is necessary while in and maintaining a position, but also while moving. Balance is often only thought of in reference to being upright, but balance reactions and responses are apparent from the very earliest stages of development. Both sitting and being on all fours are examples of balancing while maintaining a position. Crawling, walking, hopping, and jumping are examples of balancing while moving. An infant needs to be able to control its balance very early on to smoothly roll from their side onto their back and from their stomach onto their back, as there are aspects connected to the balance system and to the reactions of falling when moving between these positions. Throughout all the early developmental movement phases, we can observe the need to be able to use the body to balance in all positions and transitions (Gage et al., 2009; Bainbridge-Cohen, 1994; Feldenkrais, 1981, 1949; Hadders-Algra & Carlberg, 2008).

In Figure 3.1 we see the child go from standing to sitting, demonstrating aspects of control, tone, and balance.

Already in photo a), it can be seen that the child is in motion, managing their balance in standing. The arms are up above the height of the shoulders, with the head going backward and the hip joints bent backward.

In photo b) the child is clearly beginning to fall backward. The arms go forward and more to the sides, the head comes forward, and the hip joints bend more and go further backward. The knees bend and the fronts of both feet begin to lift from the floor.

In photo c) the child's pelvis moves farther backward and down to the floor as the head moves farther forward along with the trunk. There is a clear motion of the entire trunk from the hip joints, with the pelvis going backward and the head forward. The arms and hands move in the direction of the floor in a continuous motion, with the fingers spread open, as the child's pelvis comes down to the floor.

In photo d), the child comes with their back, head, and arms to an unsupported sitting position. This indicates that the movement of falling backward is complete, and the child comes to rest in a sitting position with their head upright.

In photos c) and d), it is noticeable that the lower back is curved backward and the mid-upper back is curved forward, reflecting an organization of the spine seen in developmental stages.

During the entire movement of going from standing to sitting by losing balance and falling backward, the child does not stiffen their arms or close their fingers, does not close their eyes or mouth. It can be seen from the child's facial expression that they experience no anxiety or fear during the motion of falling down to a sitting position on the ground. There is no reaction of the flexor muscles to falling, but rather an organized, spontaneously controlled movement, with smooth balance adaptation and fluid tone.

Turning the focus to special needs children, there may be challenges in any one of the four primary components, in a combination of two or three, or in all four to varying degrees. A child may have good control over their musculature, possess sufficient tone and balance, but have challenges in planning actions. Another child may have good ability to plan, an ability to balance, but may face obstacles related to control of movement, with the muscle tone being too high or too low. A third child may be able to plan and have the potential to control and balance, but their muscle tone is either too high or too low. Another may be able to plan and control but not have sufficient balance when beginning to move, and this may also be coupled with muscle tonus that is either too high or too low.

CASE EXAMPLE JONATHAN—STOP FOR A MOMENT, WAIT, AND ...

There are special needs children who are very verbal and possess good cognitive understanding abilities. Jonathan was such a child. He loved to talk, tell stories, and explain all sorts of things whenever we met for his sessions. Jonathan was fluent in three languages and would continuously go back and forth between them. He would very often correct my pronunciation of certain words, as I am not a native European. His vocal capacity was extraordinary. Jonathan had an understanding of what he wanted to do. He could follow any of the ideas presented to him and could plan out the ideas suggested. However, in the primary component of control, Jonathan had great difficulties. His movements were very erratic, usually fast and jerky, and executed with a lot of force and strength. He was usually patient with himself but would sometimes get frustrated at not being able to accomplish what he had in mind and wanted to do. While I was working with him, he would very often move rapidly from one topic to the next while talking, one minute saying he wanted one toy and the next saying he didn't; one moment wanting to do one thing, the next moment not wanting to anymore. One minute his answer would be, 'yes,' the next it would be, 'no.' I began to notice that his shifting back and forth between 'yes' and 'no' and his racing from one idea to the next were clearly correlated with the very fast and erratic uncontrollable shifts in his movements. Moreover, if I tried to pin him down to a clear 'yes' or 'no' answer, his movements would become even more erratic and speed up, increasing his frustration.

I am often skeptical about such simple 1:1 correlations, but exploring this one seemed to be worth a try. The safest positions and those from which he could move around by himself to some degree at his phase of development were on either his back, side, or stomach. He was familiar with these positions and could find ways to move, but could never remain still and would repeat the same movements and directions of movement over and over again without change. I felt that I needed to find a situation in movement in which he could gain control over his erratic movements so they would not 'take over him.' My assumption was that if I put him in a situation where one of the strong large muscle groups would begin to become unusable, he would not have the strength to move himself and the overall level of movement would decrease and come to a stop.

I constructed a situation for Jonathan in which his flexor muscles (which are very powerful and strong) could not move him in any direction. As always, I needed to make certain that the position would not cause him any discomfort. This can destroy the trust that has been built up and entails the risk of a child not wanting to come back or becoming uncooperative. Learning is best accomplished in an easy-going, comfortable, safe, and trusting environment. Thus, the position would have to be comfortable while simultaneously fulfilling the stipulated conditions. A short time after putting Jonathan into the position, his erratic, uncontrollable movements slowed down and then stopped completely.

At the same moment this happened, Jonathan started to talk with me, and the conversation took on a clear, deliberate 'one-way' direction. After keeping him in this very unusual position for a few moments, I brought him up to sitting in a cross-legged fashion. He became absolutely still. The look in his eyes was one of wonder. There was a subtle but clear twinkle in his eyes, and his serene peacefulness transformed the entire room. All of this took place during a demonstration in front of a large group. The stillness spread throughout the room; it was very clear to everyone in the room that this moment of stillness was precious for this young boy. From this place of stillness, he was able to sense and feel where any jerky movement that he did not intend would begin. This was a starting point, a new beginning, and a direction of learning for Jonathan. He could now feel as well as understand that he had found a way to begin to plan and control his movements.

3.3   The importance of the sensation of awkwardness

The number and types of movements that we use in daily life and in our weekly routine of activities are more or less set, e.g., the way we get out of bed to sit and stand up, the way we dress, how we sit down to eat or work, how we get into a car, the types of sports or hobbies we practice. Each activity has a specific set of routinized movements. We can do what we want to do with no great struggle or extra attention to the task at hand, indeed, without even thinking about it. It is unrehearsed and has a sensation of being ordinary.

Understand the special sensorimotor needs: It is difficult to imagine or understand what it would be like to feel awkward or clumsy in any of our routine daily activities, or to not have the means to accomplish or understand what we wish to do. However, an appreciation of these sensations is paramount to being able to begin to enter the world of sensation and learning that a special needs child—who is atypically developing and challenged—is faced with every day in their activities and therapeutic learning situations (Hanson, 1958; Feldenkrais, 1981; Edelman, 2006). They feel unable to do what it is they want to or what is asked of them. They have a sensation of awkwardness, of being clumsy, inelegant, or ungraceful. They may have no image of what they need to do to accomplish a particular activity. To an outsider, these actions may often seem very simple to perform. It can be hard to comprehend and appreciate why the child is simply not able to do it or what they experience while trying. To help convey some kind of approximating experience—one that possibly parallels the type of experience the special needs child has—I create movement situations for adults to experience what I call a sensation of awkwardness.

The movement situations comprise a specific motion pattern or one singular movement that can be clearly understood but cannot be easily done, if indeed it can be done at all. In adults, the experience is that the body does not comply with what they want it to do. People begin to move in very clumsy, uncoordinated ways. Usually, the participants either begin to giggle or show frustration. Some give up quickly, and some keep trying harder and harder, forcing themselves more and more. I tell them that this is one of the most important experiences they can have. It is one more of the building blocks required to in some way grasp a part of the sensorimotor world of a special needs child. If one wants to begin to have a wider comprehension of that which a special needs child may possibly experience on a day-to-day basis, then the experience of *not* being able to do what you want to do is important.

Personal self-learning: 'I know what to do, but I just can't make my body do it!,' 'I don't know why my body doesn't do what I want,' 'I am trying to have my body do what I want, but it does something else no matter how hard I try.' The sensation is one of 'I feel awkward, uncoordinated, and clumsy,' and it is a critical experience to have.

This is a turning point for many people. It allows them to engage with and enter into the realm of personal self-learning—its central features, constituents, and characteristics—and to appreciate its great value. Once this is accomplished, another fundamental element of the foundation for transferring and applying the ideas of early developmental movements of typically developing children to atypically developing children is in place.

Try it yourself—feeling awkward

Movement exploration:

- Find a comfortable place to lie down on your back. Bend your knees and place both of your feet on the floor. Have your knees and feet shoulder-width apart. Begin to lift the big toe of your right foot off the floor. At the same time, curl the other four toes down toward the floor and underneath your foot. Then lift the four toes and curl your big toe down and underneath your foot. Do this at least ten times.
- Notice whether you begin to do something with your mouth or one or both of your hands at the same time. Does the movement happen simply? Or do you find that when doing it, you do all sorts of unnecessary

movements that are not related to the lifting and curling? Now try the same thing with your left foot. Is it the same? More difficult?

- Now try it with both feet at the same time. Pay attention to whether each foot does something different. After trying it with both feet at the same time, straighten both your legs and take a short break. With your legs straight, turn your right leg so that all five toes face the ceiling.
- Stay in this position and begin to do the same movement of lifting the big toe, while simultaneously curling the other four toes underneath your foot and then lifting the four toes and curling your big toe underneath. Notice if your way of doing this is more difficult than when you had your feet on the floor and knees to the ceiling. After doing it ten times with your right foot, do the same ten times with your left foot and then with both feet at the same time.
- Did you at any time want to look down at your feet to see what you were doing, or try to help yourself by looking with your eyes?
- Notice the sensation of awkwardness, the sensation that you clearly understand what is being asked of you, but your body just does not do it the way you want it to and understand that it has to be done.
- On your stomach, have your lower legs bent at the knees with the bottom of your feet in the direction of the ceiling. Have your head in a comfortable position on the floor, without looking toward your feet.
- Move the big toe of one of your feet in the direction of the floor and curl the toes upward in the direction of the ceiling, and then do the opposite. Separate the big toe from the other four toes by moving the four toes in the direction of the floor and curling the big toe down toward the sole of your foot. After doing each foot separately, do both feet together and alternately. Notice the sensation and experience whether any aspect of the movement is accompanied by a sensation of awkwardness.
- Once this is complete, return to lie on your back with your legs straight and pay attention to the sensation in your feet and legs—is it any different to usual? Then stand up and take note of any differences in the sensation of standing and walking.

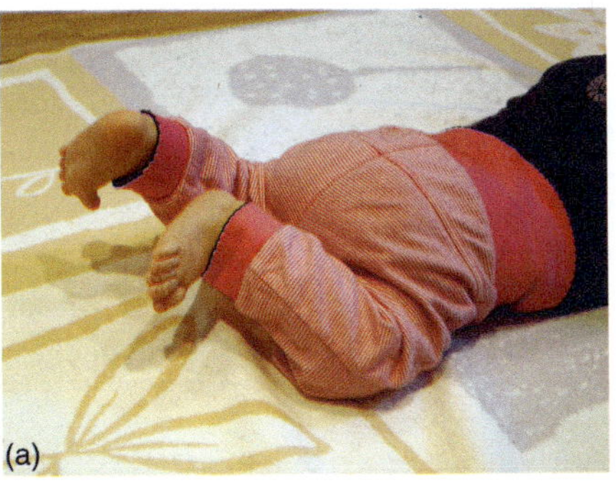
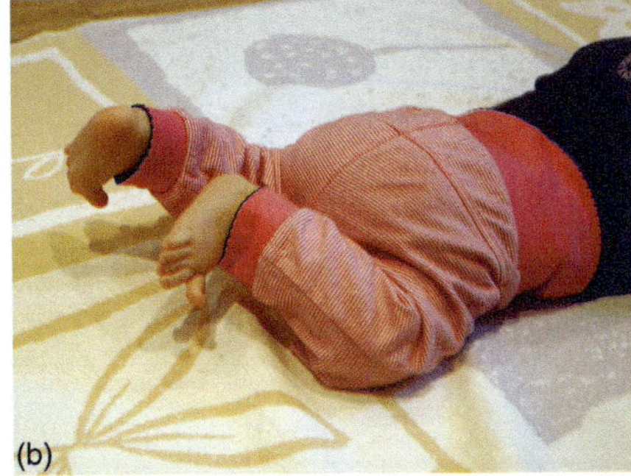

(a)   (b)

Figure 3.2: Feeling awkward

In the photos in Figure 3.2, we see an example of a child on their stomach with their knees and feet bent, using their big toe separately from the other four toes. This is a visual example of the movement exploration in the main text performed on the stomach.

In photo a), the big toe of the left foot is lifted and separated from the other four toes; on the right foot, all five toes are together.

In photo b), the big toes of both feet are lifted and separated from the other four toes.

After looking at the photos and reading the above guide to observing the photos, try once again to lie down on the floor and execute the movement exploration on your stomach.

Developmental perspectives   **4**

Movement development can be understood as a form of action intelligence, and action intelligence can, in turn, be promoted by movement development. Activity on all sensory channels (and the kinesthetic sense is the first to develop) supports learning and development in general. During *progressive developmental abilities formation*, the focus is on a motoric understanding of how a movement sequence works and how the positional transitions can be accomplished and dynamically varied.

An action network develops spontaneously, randomly, and systematically. These neuronal movement networks create increasingly complex organized movement sequences and complement each other to generate yet more. This successful transition from chaos to order characterizes a healthy, vital, and strong neuromuscular system.

Movement sequences developing in this way include

- maintaining positions, e.g., lying on your stomach with raised head, different sitting positions, standing on all fours, or standing upright, and
- deliberate transitions from one position to another.

These types of movement patterns enable dynamic reaction and adaptation to change and can be varied.

4.1 Action intelligence—understanding the world

Different forms of intelligence: Understanding through movement gives confidence. Being able to understand and figure out something new in movement gives a sense of 'I did it!'—'It was me who figured it out.' 'It *is* me!' Eureka comes in many forms, and any form of understanding

DOI: 10.4324/9781003737988-4

and knowledge is a legitimate form of intelligence. Intelligence cannot be assessed by one means only or through one lens of evaluation. The most accepted means for scoring intelligence is using a cognitive value scale. Many means have been developed to evaluate this aspect of intelligence, including its value and for what it is of value. We appraise and give this form of intelligence its value according to how we determine the rate at which the child needs to progress in order to adapt and manage particular aspects of life to attain independence and fit into society as a whole.

This is certainly one form of intelligence and one way of measuring a certain kind of intelligence. However, when looking at and contemplating unique brains, such as those of special needs children, what are our means of evaluating their particular intelligence? And how does this determine our direction for helping an individual to develop their particular kind of intelligence?

Discovering how to do something new: If we can find ways to access the child through the domain of movement in a way that allows the child to begin to figure things out for themselves, then we are effectively helping them to develop new knowledge and intelligence (Feynman, 1999). This occurs each time something new is accomplished, figured out, or actively explored by the child with curiosity. The child is then using their brain in the way all human brains function, by finding out how something new is done as an active process of discovery. This begins to foster neurological connections with the potential to bind together. When any new neurological binding takes place, it leads to new action and can be considered as new knowledge. It can be called *action intelligence*. It is new and a novel connection that did not exist previously. This is how miracles happen—this is the domain of miracles! The moments when action intelligence appears are miracle moments (see Chapter 5.5).

Wanting to find a solution: Finally being able to figure out something that was elusive or solving something that was unfeasible are qualities we value. What is it that drives the figuring out and solving process? What motivates and pushes the child to solve something? Is the drive and motivation to figure things out a general human quality? If yes, then we need to find situations to challenge special needs children to promote this. This wakes up a part of the child's brain and stimulates the human drive to find solutions, to want to know.

The action intelligence in the figuring out process is in the how to do something, how to accomplish the action. There is movement and there is turning a movement into an action. The engagement in the *how of the doing* is the child being actively engaged in their own learning and development—whether they know it or not (Figure 4.1).

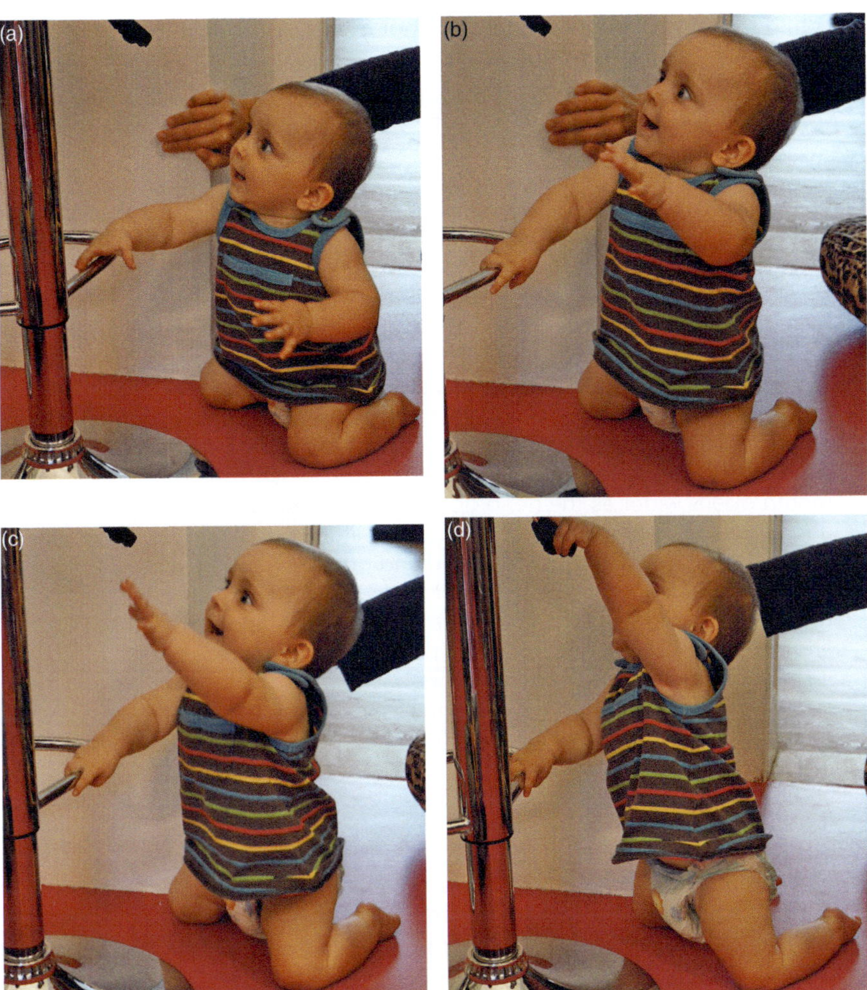

Figure 4.1: Experiencing action intelligence

Action understanding: Being engaged in the act of figuring out does not necessarily imply cognitive understanding of what has been figured out in the standard sense. However, if this leads to any new form of action and doing, then it can be said that there is action understanding. What was figured out opens up a new way to do something in a developing child; it means that a new movement—any new movement in any child, whether typically or atypically developing—will help to create a cascade of new possibilities and connections. It is always important to remember that there is no single way to do this. No one way to help the child break through to this flow of development. The proof that the path taken with the child was the right one is the child's accomplishments. This does not exclude outside interventions that are sometimes needed to allow these directions to continue. These outside interventions remove roadblocks that cannot be got around by learning alone.

In the photo sequence in Figure 4.1, we can observe the movement of a child done with curiosity, motivation, and intention. The process shows the child's action intelligence and illustrates the how of doing the movement.

In photo a), the child is gazing wide-eyed at the black handle on the stool. The right hand is in the process of taking hold of the stool's lower bar, as observed in the thumb and index finger. The child's left hand is in an open-fingered anticipatory reaching configuration; their head is held with the chin away from the throat and the back extended.

In photo b), the fingers of the right hand begin to come more clearly around the bar of the stool, as the left arm and hand begin to reach forward and upward in the direction of the handle focused on by the eyes. The mouth opens wider as the head goes slightly further backward. The pelvis and upper legs move forward and upwards, lifting out of the initial position.

In photo c), the weight of the head and trunk begins to shift to the right as the arm lifts higher, and the hand and fingers show a clear direction toward the back bar of the stool. The fingers of the right hand close more around the lower bar, as seen in the position of the thumb.

In photo d), the head moves farther backward, with the back extending and the pelvis pushing forward as the arm reaches upward. The weight of the head and trunk continues to shift to the right as the child reaches their intended goal of the black handle.

All elements of the execution of the intended action are coordinated in the movement—planning, control, balance, and timing. It is a functional movement directed by the child's interest in figuring out how to reach the object of its curiosity. The muscular strength needed to reach up and push the pelvis forward and up over the knees is present at this developmental stage and assists the child in realizing its intention.

CASE EXAMPLE BARBARA—OUTSIDE THE COMFORT ZONE

Barbara is an extraordinarily intelligent verbal child with a smile that melts you in seconds. She has a strong will and desire to learn and progress, and is not prepared to let her cerebral palsy get in the way of what she wants to do or define who she is or wants to be. Barbara used a walker to help maintain balance in standing, and she would bring her walker with her to sessions.

For certain children, using a walker can be an end goal; for others, it represents a mode of transition to independent walking. For Barbara, it was neither: it was a bothersome and annoying impediment. Having a child get to know their walker and use it not just for walking can be an important learning tool. The walker is a part of them for many hours a day, and it is good for them to become familiar with it and be able to use it in a versatile way. If the walker can become familiar enough that they can also use it in a fun, active, and creative way, then it ceases to be an impediment or a bother and becomes a useful partner in daily life. This was one goal of the work with Barbara.

This manner of thinking was gleaned through the example of my father. My father lost one of his legs in an accident at the age of three, when he was run over by a streetcar. This did not stop him from excelling in sports and becoming captain of the gymnastics team in high school. He became the state champion in parallel bars and rings. When he was up in the air on the rings or the bars, the floor was no longer an impediment to him; he was freed of the floor's constraints. His balance until the end of his life was impeccable. Sometimes his stump would swell, and he would not be able to wear his prosthesis for a week or two. He had to use crutches until it had healed. He would often show how he could play and do all sorts of tricks on his crutches: handstands on the crutches, twirling around, hopping and skipping, going from one crutch to the other—all with only one leg to use.

He was the master of his crutches; they were a tool he could use however he wished and not just as they were designed to be. His creativity in the use of his crutches at these times left an indelible memory. For him they were not crutches but an object he could transform into something interesting, disconnected from their intended purpose. This provides great inspiration when working with children in walkers or wheelchairs and forms the basis of a creative thinking model.

One of the first tasks with Barbara was to help her to sense and feel the movements done together in sessions, so she could begin to recognize more easily where she needed to improve aspects of her balance and walking.

A big issue for Barbara was feeling comfortable in situations where she needed to balance on her own. She had her repertoire of what she knew and recognized in sitting, getting up out of a chair, standing, and walking, and felt she didn't need to learn any other ways. To improve their balance, many children with cerebral palsy need to have their balance challenged and disturbed before any significant progress takes place. This needs to be outside of the 'comfort zone' they have become used to, know well, and are comfortable with, but still in a relatively safe situation where they can manage themselves and not become overwhelmed. Losing balance without having the means to recover it can be very frightening for anyone, let alone for a young child with cerebral palsy who has not yet developed a great balance ability and constantly faces challenging situations. If new perturbations are offered in small increments, then balance can be increasingly challenged and begin to improve.

However small the challenges and disturbances are, they need to be offered in a way that is surprising to the child and which they do not expect at first. This requires the use of different rhythms and speeds and playing with the child's expectations. The reason is that to regain lost balance when you are prepared for it is not so difficult, but the true improvement comes from situations where the response and the reaction need to be very fast, automatic, and spontaneous. The child needs to learn to tolerate the sensation of being out of control and to trust their own body and its response.

Barbara needed to start in a chair and learn to come out of the chair and up to standing in a number of different ways. When the speed was varied unexpectedly, she just stopped and protested. She folded her arms over her chest and simply refused to cooperate. Barbara was no longer the smiling little girl that everyone recognized, but a stubborn, defiant child. With her arms crossed over her chest and her head hanging down, she made a very serious, defiant face and began to say very loudly over and over again in her native language, 'I don't want to!' She would then gaze over at her mother and repeat over and over again, 'I don't want to! I won't! I won't! I won't!'

Whenever a new challenge is introduced to a child, one should never be taken aback by the child's initial responses and behaviors. If the child trusts you and senses that you are there to help them, they will eventually go along with you, provided you 'accompany' rather than force them and are completely present with the child. Barbara's 'I don't want to!' was uttered any time a new demand and challenge to her balance was introduced. She knew she could rise to the challenge and would succeed, but it demanded great inner strength and courage each time. Whenever beginning, when Barbara sensed that something new was coming, she immediately crossed her arms, stopped, and protested.

It was so impressive that Barbara never said, 'I can't!' but always, 'I don't want to!' It was her way of saying, 'I know I need to do this, and it is good for me, and I will be pleased with myself when I do it, but I am happy where I am!' 'Can't I just stay here where I am?' As adults, we learn to cope with and manage such demands and challenges, but for a 4-year-old, this represents an extraordinary feat of maturity—emotional and intellectual.

Once Barbara had experienced a few successes and surmounted her fears and legitimate wariness of the challenges and difficulties of the new movements and sensations, she was fine. It was not just fine each time she finally succeeded, but there were also miraculous and magical moments for Barbara in her inner experience and in the sharing of this sensation of herself with others around her. She became more and more courageous, and not only did she stop crossing her arms and saying, 'I don't want to!' but transformed it into, 'Don't help me; I can do it on my own!' 'What is the next thing you have for me to try?' 'Let's keep going!' It actually became possible to tease her about how she had behaved at first and how far she had come.

Behaviors and attitudes such as Barbara's show the nature of the human spirit and the courage of such extraordinary children in light of the objective challenges they face day in and day out. To bear witness to these moments and how the children rise to meet the situations is always moving. Barbara improved enormously and learned to balance in so many different situations; she would use her walker in a way that reminded me of my father with his crutches.

4.2 Progressive developmental abilities formation

Models of movement development: The past few hundred years have seen a variety of models of movement development. The theories behind some models were based solely on observation, whereas others considered the science of the time, asked questions from that perspective, and related them to infants' movement development (Piek, 2006).

Some models focus exclusively on movement and others focus more on the child's overall behavior, including emotional, social, and environmental relationships. The theories all have ramifications for practical application of the models when working with typically and atypically developing children. Over the past 100 years, the prevalent model has been the milestones model. This model focuses on looking at what the infant and baby should be doing in which positions and during which timeframe. In milestones and many of the other models, there is no in-depth discussion of the way in which the child does the movement, how the baby arrives at doing a particular movement, or how they come to be in a position or leave it for another. There is also very little, if any, discussion of the components and building blocks required for learning the movements and positions of a milestone, or of the specifics and variety involved in its make-up.

Progressive developmental abilities formation: A model of movement development needs to account for the changes that take place and are seen in the variety of movement positions and transitions, along with the abilities and skills that develop during and as a result of these movements.

The model should encompass the *processes* and *mechanisms* that are involved in helping these changes in movements, positions, and skills evolve.

An appropriate model needs to consider not only which position but also the how of arriving at the position, the possible variety of ways of moving out of a position, and the intra- and interdynamics of learning to be in and remain in a position. This is also applicable to transitional movements, e.g., rolling, coming from the stomach to sitting, or crawling.

In shaping my ideas, I intended to fashion a model that would be open yet defined by a clear framework with room to include diverse outlooks. What resulted was the model of *progressive developmental abilities formation*: an open yet well-defined framework allowing for clear application and direction of ideas. The model takes into account not only the child but also their social and physical surroundings. It provides direction, a definition of what is in process, and the goals that can be achieved.

Progressive developmental abilities formation

Progressive: Progress, advancement, and improvement are sought. This defines the need to stride forward, not getting stuck in one place or just being in the process. The aim is advancement toward a goal, becoming better and improving, with continuity and realization of positive change.

Developmental: The primary phases and stages of the child in terms of the development of movement, sensation, emotion, and cognition. The child's relationships to themself, others, and the outside world. All aspects of movement leading up to standing, walking, hopping, skipping, and jumping.

Abilities: Abilities are the dynamic component of what we look for when viewing a growing young child. In essence, we do not look for what the child can, should, or will do; we rather view the ability the child needs or has in order to be able to do what they do. We see the ability as a large form of action and the child's reactions to their experience of themself as well as their physical and social environment. Ability encompasses the entirety of a child. The main medium in which to view the progress and development of abilities that are achieved is movement.

Formation: Formation is the materialization and manifestation of a developmental ability or abilities as a solid structure or active pattern that is predictable, repeatable, and dependable. The child's early evolving age- and growth-related elements of movement and developmental abilities establish themselves solidly and clearly; they manifest and materialize in a particular form. The abilities and movements form clear configurations and a stable yet dynamic organization. For children, the formation of an ability includes the possibility to continuously improve. To name an example: when a child learns to walk, after the first one or two weeks during which they only take a few successive steps, we continue to observe changes in the way the child walks for many months and even years, while the formed ability continues to further develop into skipping, hopping, jumping, and running.

The model of *progressive developmental abilities formation* provides clear direction and a wide range of possibilities for practical application with a goal in mind, while respecting the learning processes needed by the child. We seek progress in the child's early developmentally evolving abilities, and work toward these arranging themselves in a clear form of behavior and action.

4.3 Development of movement patterns—random, organized, systematic

Neural movement networks form and combine to create patterns of more and more complex organized movement. Creating order out of a chaotic and disorganized neuromuscular system is a quality of a healthy, vigorous, and strong system.

4.3.1 Random exploration

In a typically developing child, the various physiological systems that organize movement have an enormous variety of neuromusculoskeletal possibilities and variations at their disposal. During the first months of life, an infant spends much of their time immersed in exploratory movements (Thelen & Smith, 1994). The child performs the movements smoothly and seamlessly using a large variety of configurations and combinations, and does so over an extended period of time (Figure 4.2). During a later phase in the first year, the child begins to engage in and explore more task-oriented movements, activities, and behaviors. For an infant in the early period of random exploratory movements, the greater the variety of movements available to explore, the better. The more movement configurations, combinations, and directions the infant has in their initial repertoire, the more they will have to select from later for efficient and effective patterns of action, behavior, and engagement. This diversity helps the infant to find the most appropriate and effective ways of adapting to new situations they encounter. Through this process of exploration of novel combinations, the child acquires innovative ways to move in and through their physical environment and interact with situations in the surrounding social world. Following this initial exploratory phase, the infant begins to develop ways to use these variations and combinations for intentional voluntary actions and interactions.

The neuromuscular system of a special needs child often does not have this opportunity to engage in a wide range of exploratory movements. It may have a reduced variety of possible movements to begin with, as well as a reduced means to explore and combine these movement possibilities.

Looking at this property of growth and development from the perspective of therapeutic learning, it is useful to think about how to find specific ways to help a special needs child's neuromuscular system experience a process of exploration of movement combinations and variations. When

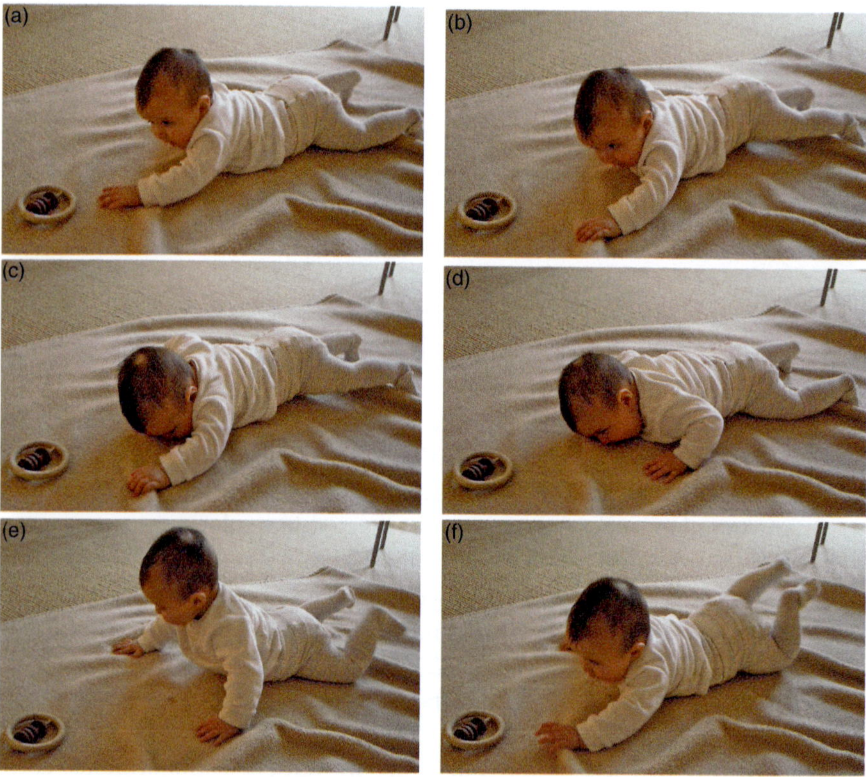

Figure 4.2: Combining movement elements

variations are presented to the special needs child along with numerous ways to combine them, it becomes more probable that the child will form new patterns of movement in their actions, behaviors, and emotions. The process of the child being able to try out novel movement patterns either by themself or under guidance is of great value for growth and development of the child's neuromusculoskeletal system. Additional variations of movements and novel ways to combine these movements are needed to elaborate and expand the developmental repertoire (Hadders-Algra & Carlberg, 2008; Hüther, 2018; Stergiou & Decker, 2011). As a result, the child will arrive at a richer personal experience of themselves—by means similar to those of a typically developing system—of their own accord and without any prompting.

It is important to understand how these combinations and variations should be offered and presented to the child to aid the process of forming a network of stable and useful movement patterns.

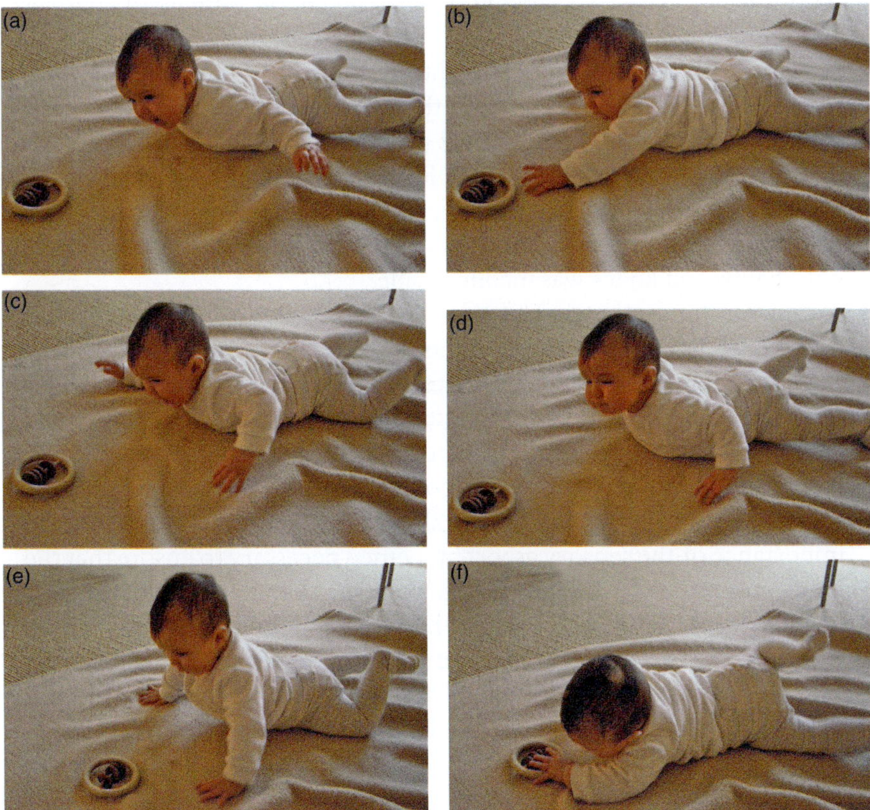

Figure 4.3: Combining movement elements

The experience of new exploratory variations in movement is also relevant for adults. As adults, we have formed routines and established preferences for certain ways of moving. These patterns were often learned very early in life and were effective adaptations at the time. However, later in life, our earlier adaptations and preferences may no longer be as efficient as they once were. These preferences can be discovered by trying out new combinations and variations of movement that do not belong to our usual daily repertoire. Through exploring and discovering new ways of moving, we can become mindful of our routines; we can freely choose that which works best for us at a particular stage of life, and not remain stuck in our habits.

CASE EXAMPLE ALAN—TAKING PRIDE IN ONE'S OWN REPERTOIRE OF MOVEMENTS

Alan was not even 1.5 years old. He had a general stiffness of muscles and joints in all parts of his body. When placed on his back he would lie with his legs completely straight, with his head lifted off the floor and looking down toward his feet the entire time. Alan did not do any transitional movements, and it was nearly impossible to put him in any developmental positions, let alone for him to maintain a position if he could be brought into it. It was difficult for him to open or bend his legs, or to move his arms and bring them over his head. Sitting or coming onto hands and knees was inconceivable.

During the first period of Alan's sessions, the primary focus was to begin to have all the major joints and muscle groups able to move. It was imperative that he begin to have experiences and sensations of moving in all the possible basic directions on his back, side, and stomach. Without the joints and muscles going into and through these basic varieties of movements and configurations, he really had no basis for sensation of his joints or, naturally, the movements. Coupled to the importance of the sensory aspect, it seemed necessary to ensure that the joints and muscles could do the movements voluntarily or that it was possible for someone else to move him through them with their hands. The thinking behind this was that if the joints and muscle groups could gain flexibility and Alan's sensory domain would open up as a result, then there would be a chance that his abilities might begin to emerge.

Extreme care was necessary to find the easiest direction of movement for each and every joint. Progress was slow at first, and the movements and directions presented to Alan had to be precise, systematic, and orderly. All the movements required many repetitions. Yet, once all the basic directions of the joints and muscle groups began to become fluid, significant changes started to appear.

The first was being able to bring Alan into a sitting position in a variety of ways, and his being able to maintain the position. This led to him being able to follow almost any direction proposed to him to come into sitting. The joy in the parents' eyes the first times he sat on his own for a few seconds was highly memorable. Slowly but surely, it was possible to assist Alan to sit unaided with his legs crossed and in a side-sitting position, and to sit with his lower legs hanging off the table with his back and head upright.

The next stage was to find ways to have Alan come onto his hands and knees, and also up onto his knees without having his hands on the floor. Alan still could not do any of these transitional movements by himself. He always needed very clear assistance and hands-on guidance.

Alan was nonverbal, and when he first started his sessions, he was not particularly expressive. As time went on and his movement repertoire increased, his expression began to emerge. In each session, Alan could now be moved through many transitional sequences and into many positions. As the fluidity of his movements improved, a decision had to be made regarding whether to try and use the time to find a way to make all the basic movement transitions on his back, side, stomach, to sitting, and onto his knees become voluntary, or to keep the movement progression in the direction of standing and walking as the priority. As he was now very flexible and could recognize all the movement directions proposed and suggested to him using hands-on guidance, it became apparent that he had enough muscular strength to bring himself up to standing. He was also old enough now to introduce him to walking. There was no reason to wait.

The expression on Alan's face when he was brought to standing for the first time was indescribable. He was filled with pride and joy. To be present in his moment of joyfulness and see how he shared it with his parents was a gift—his elation filled the room, and he expressed it with his whole being and in very loud, jubilant vocalization! He was stable and movable on his feet, and ready to try steps. His response was immediate, and he took step after step in the direction of his parents. Walking is one of the prime goals of development. There are many health benefits for any child to be up and movable in standing and walking. There is never a need to wait to bring a child up to standing and walking when they have the strength. This gives abilities that are unique to the standing position in space the chance to emerge and develop. Alan was a good example of this. All earlier developmental movement positions and transitions are aided by standing upright and walking.

4.3.2 Systematic action networks

An action network develops spontaneously, randomly, and systematically. Spontaneity in action is when a particular movement or action is not planned. Randomness is when a movement occurs in an arbitrary manner. Systematically is when an event is focused, consistent, and methodically performed.

Spontaneity and randomness: These are key elements seen in the development and formation of movement and action networks in very young, typically developing children. Development of a movement and action network also follows a very clear order. This order is created by the baby's spontaneously and randomly performed movements and their interaction with the social and physical environment. At the same time, spontaneity, randomness, and order have a clear, well-defined form. The form is the combination of the particular movement elements in a random order. When these random combinations are performed by the child, they are done so spontaneously.

System and repetition: The systematic performance of spontaneous, randomly ordered movements creates a spontaneous randomly organized movement combination. When this is repeated numerous times, each repetition uses the same movement elements, whereby these elements are combined and performed in a slightly different manner and/or order (Figure 4.3). In this way, a network begins to form. Further repetitions employing different parts of the body in different configurations assist in forming more networks.

The photo sequences in Figures 4.2 and 4.3 are thematically connected. They are examples of movements done spontaneously, randomly, and systematically. In both sequences, the child uses the same elements of movement but combines them differently while focusing on and attempting to reach the ring in front of them. At this stage, the child does not have the ability for forward locomotion on the stomach. The intention is the same; the attempts to realize the intention use different combinations of the same elements.

In Figure 4.2, photo a), the child looks toward the ring with their head up, legs long, knees on the floor. In photo b), the left side of the pelvis and left knee lift off the floor as the pelvis turns to the right, and the left hand

and arm come farther away from the ring. In c) the head goes down, the rest remains the same. In photo d), the left arm bends at the elbow, and the elbow comes off the floor, with the left hand coming into a position to push the floor, while the left knee and left side of the pelvis return to the floor. In e) both arms straighten, and the head and chest come away from the floor. Both knees bend, and the feet come away from the floor. In photo f), the left arm reaches out to the ring, the pelvis tilts in such a way as to arch the lower back, and the right knee comes off the floor.

In the second photo sequence, Figure 4.3, the same elements of movement are used in the same position with the same intention but combined in a different manner and order. After reading through the description of the first photo sequence, try to observe the same elements of movement in the second sequence and how they are combined differently.

4.3.3 *Organized self-learning processes*

Organization: This has practical implications for special needs children: when a child is offered and guided through movements systematically and repeatedly, the child's system begins to have a greater possibility to function in a manner similar to that of a typically developing child, which thus simulates typical neuromuscular system activity. An experiential learning developmental growth process begins to form and become more available to the child. This type of randomly systematically organized learning with a spontaneous quality brings essential elements into the child's field of experience. These types of rich experiences are those required by a thriving, typically developing system, and the system indeed depends on them.

There are very specific developmental movements that the child needs to be directed toward in this process. By design, the direction of all development is always in the direction of standing and walking. It is important to study the specific movements, types, varieties, and variations of movements that can and do combine at all the different stages of early development. This enables one to interact with an actively growing child and provide the necessary input where and when it is required. In this way, action patterns emerge and form more quickly and easily.

Self-organization, exploration of movement possibilities, and spontaneous behavior are qualities that are vital for an atypically developing child to experience, cultivate, and nurture. This provides the atypically developing child with the realistic possibility of generating active, continuous self-learning. It fosters direction and progression, helping the child to go through a multifaceted process of guided and unguided experiential self-exploration and learning that they were not able to spontaneously generate, produce, and spawn unaided. This process may have been lacking during the period of very early infancy and various other phases of growth during which the mechanisms of internally self-generated spontaneous variation of movement act. Clear application of these ideas provides tremendous freedom to work with a child and achieve very productive outcomes.

4.4   The dynamic nature of positions and transitions

A basic definition of movement is the change of something from one position to another in space. By its very meaning, movement is comprised of at least two different positions and includes the transition between them, i.e., the leaving of one position and the arrival in the other. In the stages of developmental movement learning and acquisition, both transitions and positions are very important.

4.4.1   Positions

Positions are considered to be places and locations in which the situation is stable, static, stationary, motionless, inactive, and quiet. There are no surprises or moments of uncertainty in a position. It can remain constant unless something comes along to disturb it: a very safe, stable situation which one knows, recognizes, is accustomed to, and comfortable in. When we are familiar with a particular position, we may not be so amenable to trying out another one, which would require us to leave the position we are in and move to another. Even if something comes along and tries to force us out of the position, we may try as we can not to move and stay where we are. The better we know the position, the harder it can be for us to move or be moved to another.

Examples of positions are lying on your stomach with your head raised, a variety of sitting positions, being supported on hands and knees, and standing (Figure 4.4).

The child must learn how to arrive and maintain itself in a position while tolerating varieties of perturbations which try to destabilize the position itself (Thelen & Smith, 1994, 1993; Feldenkrais, 1949; Hadders-Algra & Carlberg, 2008). There is an enormous trove of learning the child explores in forming the ability of how to arrive in a position, remain in it, and then

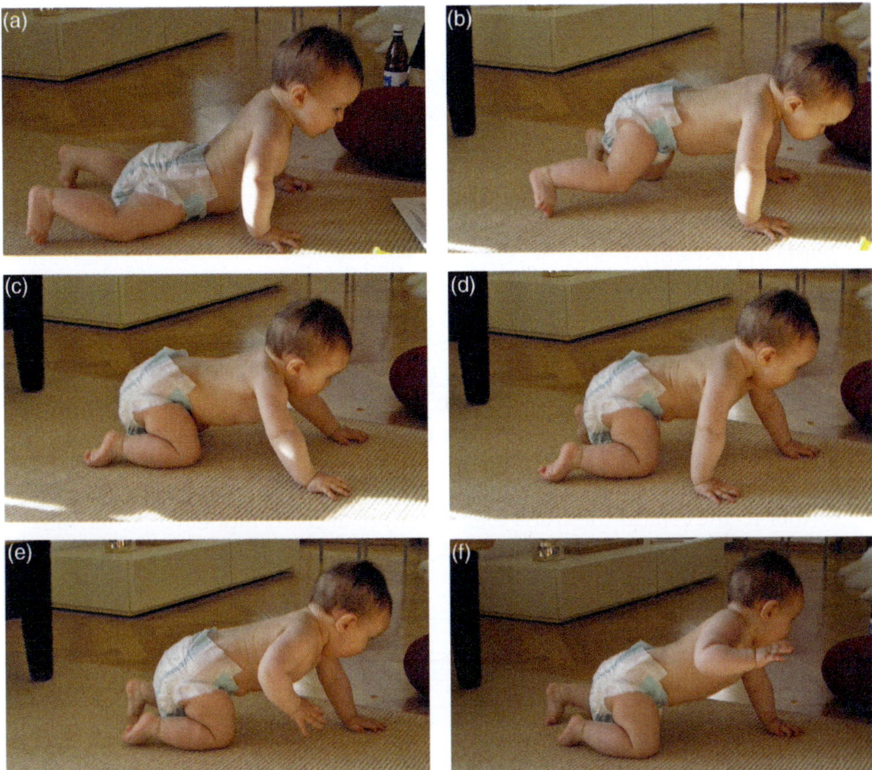

Figure 4.4: Transitional movement 1

leave it for another or return to it. In typical development, we observe that there are almost inexhaustible ways to arrive at and be in different positions and then to leave them again.

Figure 4.4 as well as the subsequent photo sequences in this chapter show a variety of different transitional and positional movements. In each of the sequences, there are noticeable transitions of weight, balance, and orientation, with movements coordinating many joints at different heights in gravity, limb adjustments to different configurations, and movements from one place to another in the environment.

In photo a), the child is supporting themself on both hands and straight arms. Their weight is directly over the shoulder joints and hands. The chest and upper part of the pelvis are off the floor, the legs are long, and the thighs and knees are in contact with the floor.

In photo b), the child has moved to supporting themself on two hands and one knee, with their chest, belly, and pelvis off the floor. The child's head is facing more toward the floor, and their weight remains directly over the shoulder joints and hands.

In photo c), the child comes to being on both knees and both hands symmetrically. The head has lifted and the weight of the body has shifted backward, with the pelvis more toward the heels and the hip joints more bent.

In photo d), the child moves to a position with asymmetrical support on their arms.

In photo e), the right arm lifts from the floor and bends at the elbow, with the right knee coming closer to the right arm. The head shifts over to the left, bringing the weight over the support of the left arm. The support remains asymmetrical on one arm, with one knee in front of the other. The left side has become longer than the right.

In photo f), the right arm is raised, and the weight of the trunk shifts further to the left, as the trunk extends more and lifts higher together with the head. The distance between the knees increases, as observed by the distance between the feet.

4.4.2 Transitions

Transitions are movements that bring us from one place to another, from one body position to another. Transitional movements are composed of combinations of elements that produce the possibility to move the entire body to a different situation through various configurations and at different heights in gravity. The movements can be very unstable and have elements of various speeds and stopping points. There is always a starting position and an end position to a transitional movement, as in rolling or coming to up sitting. To develop proficiency in transitioning, the child's neuromusculoskeletal system needs to interact with different kinds of environments and obstacles in the environment to be able to realize its intention of arriving at a particular position. Typically developing children spend hours and hours of each day experimenting with, learning, and experiencing many different ways to move from one position to another. In each and every successive attempt, they gain more knowledge and skill regarding how and what to do to arrive at a certain place and leave it again. As the first year of life progresses, the child gets higher and higher in gravity, from being on their back and stomach, all the way to standing and walking. Each new level of gravity it achieves demands that the child interact with more complex and challenging situations (Figure 4.5).

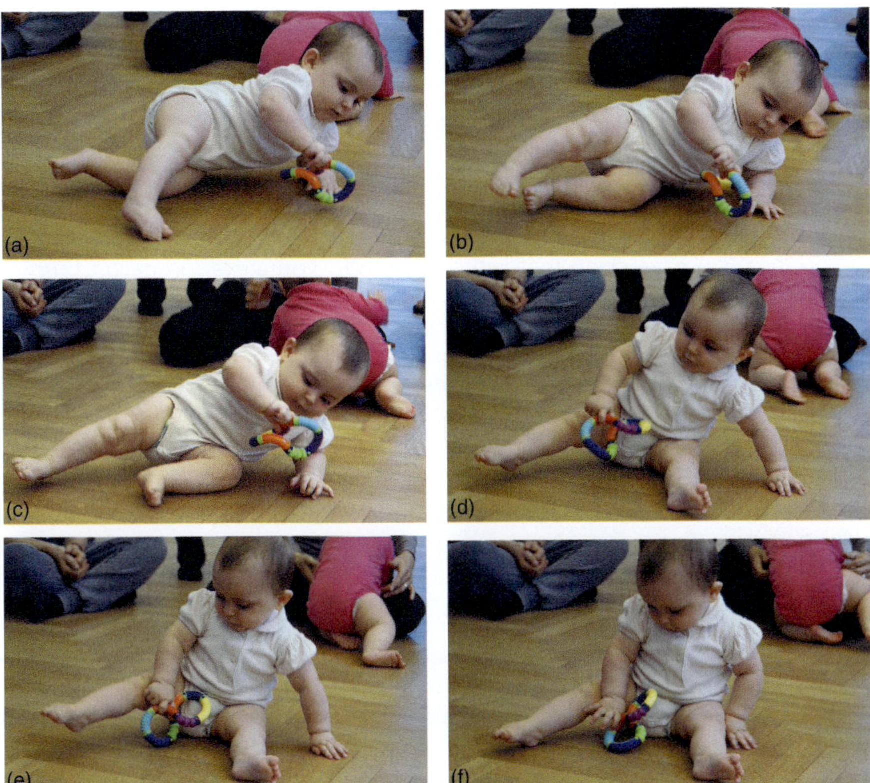

Figure 4.5: Transitional movement 2

Transitional movements

Transitional movements are structures in which the child learns to find solutions for

- transitions of weight,
- keeping balance,
- changes of orientation,
- movements coordinating many joints to move at different heights in gravity,
- limb adjustment to variations in speed in different configurations,
- moving from one place in the environment to another,
- finding how to get and take something they want, and
- learning to achieve a means to an end.

Try it yourself—positions and transitions

An example to understand the difference between a position and a transition experientially is sitting. Take a moment to write down at least five different sitting positions on the floor.

After you have written them down, get down onto the floor and put yourself into these five different positions.

Once you have done that, write down how you arrived in each of the positions and how you left them. Think of what it is that allows you to remain in any of the various sitting positions you chose and how you begin to move out of each of these positions.

Being in motion and transitioning from one position to another can be something very simple. It can also be challenging or even frightening if we cannot control the speed or the direction of any of our limbs, or if we cannot stop the movement where and when we want to (Figure 4.6).

Think of walking or driving along in the winter and, all of a sudden, you reach a patch of ice you hadn't seen or expected. You immediately lose control of both speed and directionality. How and where you may end up will be a matter of chance unless you can regain control. The sensation of speed and being out of control, not knowing where you are going or how you will be when you end up there, can be very frightening.

Another example might be the first attempt at ice skating or skiing. At the beginning, the loss of control, slipping, and sliding can make the body very stiff and contribute to falling. The fear that emerges in such situations is the innate fear of falling and its physiologic automatic response, including breath holding and stiffening of the chest, arms, and hands (Konner, 2010; Bainbridge-Cohen, 1994; Feldenkrais, 1981, 1949). Slowly, you begin to learn how to use your body in this unfamiliar situation. You figure out how to control your movement despite the ice or snow, and you gain the skills to influence the direction and speed of your movements despite the constant need to readjust. Once you have adopted and learned the reactions and responses required in such a changing dynamic situation, you begin to enjoy and actually take pleasure in the movement. The changes of speed and direction, the stopping and starting and moving around on a very unstable surface are thrilling, and the challenges of the continuous changes keep your system fresh and alert.

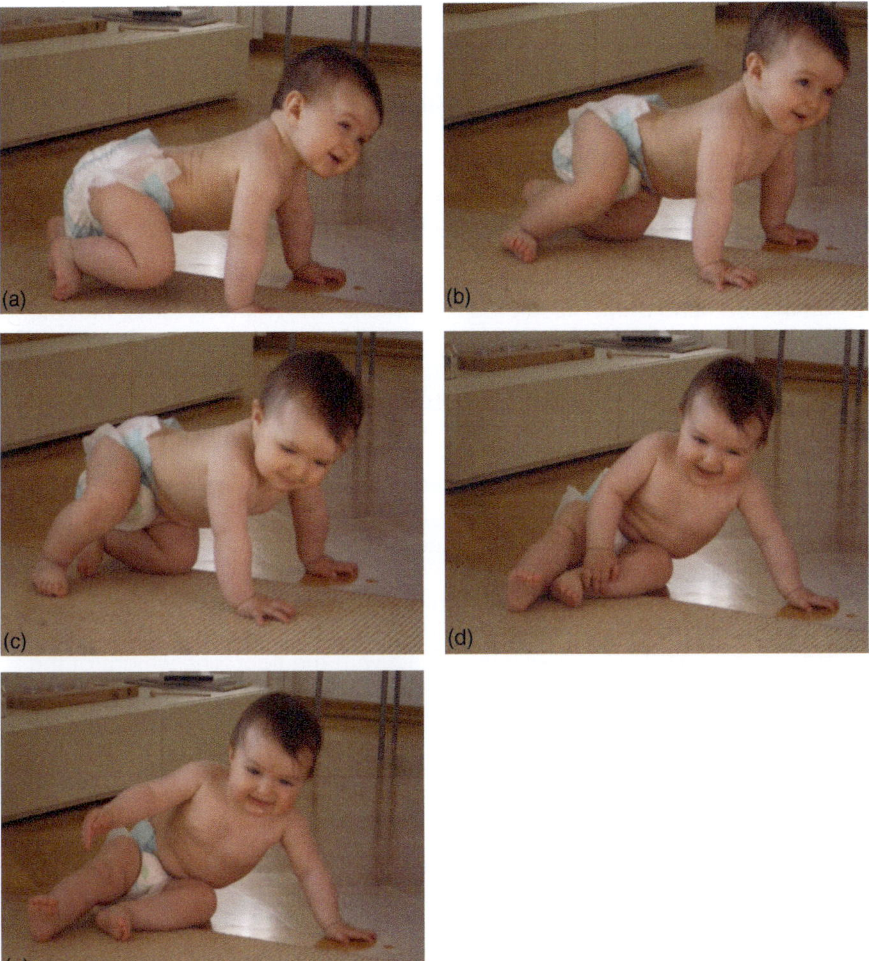

Figure 4.6: Transitional movement 3

In Figure 4.5, a transition from being on the side supported by one forearm and elbow to coming to sitting with legs outstretched can be seen. The child is holding a toy upon which its eyes are fixed the entire time as they transition to sitting.

In photo a), the child is looking at a toy they are holding in their right hand. The child leans and supports themself on the left forearm and elbow. The chest and pelvis are in the air, and there is a side-bending from the head to the pelvis, with the middle of the chest hanging toward the floor. The left leg is bent, with the foot and lower leg in the air. The right leg is stretched out in front, with the toes touching the floor and the heel in the air.

In photo b), the legs change, with the right leg pointing straight down in a continuation of the right side and the left knee bent in front of the pelvis. The forearm and elbow become visible.

In photo c), the left knee comes closer to the chest as the right leg moves closer to the floor with the right foot flexing. There is now less side-bending from the head to the pelvis on the right side.

In photo d), the left elbow comes off the floor, and the body is supported on the left hand only. The left leg straightens. The right leg turns, with the front of the foot directed toward the ceiling. This leads to tonification of the belly muscles on the right side and the front of the right leg. The head and eyes continue to remain fixed on the toy in the child's hand.

In photo e), the right arm goes down toward the floor, with the head tilting forward and also looking down at the floor.

In photo f), the transition is completed as the right foot touches the floor.

Figure 4.6 shows a transitional movement from being supported by three points—the hands and one knee—to being supported by one point, namely the left hand.

In photo a), the child is supported on both arms and the left knee.

In photo b), the weight of the child's pelvis shifts to the left as the inner side of the right foot comes into contact with the floor. The weight of the pelvis is no longer on the left knee but rather outside of the left knee, as the left upper thigh is adducted and the head moves to the right.

In photo c), the head is looking down and to the right. The visual orientation changes, the sole of the right foot comes onto the floor, and the right knee opens.

In photo d), the pelvis on the left side comes down to the floor as the right leg straightens and the right arm lifts off the floor. The weight of the body leans, supported by the left hand. This leaning allows the chest on the left side to hang and remain long.

In photo e), the movement continues as the right leg turns with the toes more to the ceiling, and the right arm continues its trajectory and lifts from the floor.

The entire body is involved in this transitional movement of bringing the pelvis to the floor while moving around the support of one arm, shoulder blade, and shoulder joint.

4.4.3 Inner dynamics of transitional and positional movements

One might be inclined to think that no movement is taking place while in a position that it is static, and, conversely, that movement is a constant feature of a transition. However, upon closer examination, it can be seen that there is a great deal of movement taking place while in a position, and there are also many stopping points during a transition. A deeper understanding of these aspects helps us to understand and clarify their use and application for learning in special needs children as well as in adults.

Dynamic reactions and changes: Being able to transition and position are learned abilities. Both are dynamic states. The dynamics are the responses, adaptations, and changes made by a child while actively learning a developmental position or transition. These dynamic responses and changes can provide insight into the individuality of each child (Thelen & Smith, 1993, 1994). No two people perform the same movement in the same way, even though the movement itself is the same, e.g., directly rolling from the floor to sitting and standing, or getting up from a chair.

Intra- and inter-movement dynamics: During learning and development of the ability to transition and position, dynamics exist both within (intra-) and between (inter-) movements. This is true in terms of a general ability as well as for specific positions and transitions. The dynamics are a collaboration between muscles, joints, and the environment, comprising subtle yet significant adjustments, reactions, and responses that allow the transition to develop, continue, and stay on track in order to reach the ultimate goal.

These dynamic transitional reactions and responses help to guide the movement toward a different end goal, or along another path if the original goal or path is disturbed along the way and cannot be reached as planned. Disturbances may be a change in the environment, perhaps a toy, pillow, piece of furniture, or a sibling coming along and interfering in some way. These intradynamics can only be seen when the movement taking place is broken down into smaller components.

Variations: When considering the intra- and interdynamics of movement positions and transitions, one needs to keep in mind both the many possible small variations and the neurobiological value to the developing brain of this variety in means of arriving, leaving, and remaining. Many points are passed along the way before a movement becomes a full transition. These incremental elements that converge to form a complete transitional movement are important and relevant. The many small variations that can represent part of any transitional movement, e.g., coming up to sitting from the stomach or back (Figure 4.7), are fundamental to know, and, moreover, they are critical in therapeutic learning situations.

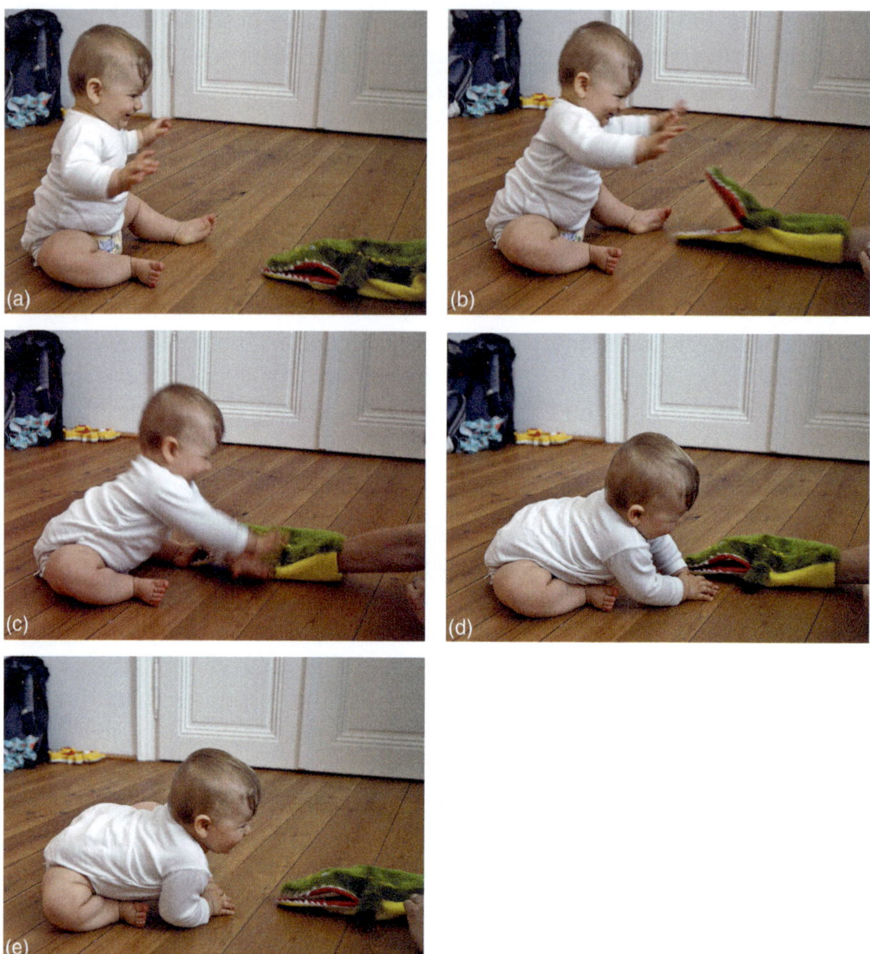

Figure 4.7: Transitional movement 4

There are intradynamics of a position that contribute to learning how to find *stability* in any given position. When observing any of the positions in which the baby arrives through their own active initiation, we can see instability and movement—a tremendous number of small movements are required for the child to learn how to become stable and remain in a position. We also see how the baby continuously adapts to changes produced by their own physical adjustments to external social or environmental perturbances. The longer the baby interacts in the position to try and remain in it, the more intradynamic movements they make. The variety and directionality of these subtle adjustments give the baby more ability to initiate leaving the position in a variety of directions and help them get to know the ways back to the positions through varieties of transitions. The more a position is 'usable' for the child—to do something, play, or be socially absorbed—the more they will form ways to minimize the sways, swings, and flows of perturbations they need to manage to remain in the position.

Exploration of possibilities for transitioning and positioning: Turning the focus to special needs children, we find the challenges they face with positioning and transitioning. The special needs child often lacks the ability to freely explore new and varied ways of transitioning and positioning. Being guided by another through the intradynamics of a transition or position assists in initiating the learning and development of a larger repertoire of transitions and positions. The child also needs to be accompanied along the path to encountering many of the types of adaptations needed to successfully experience and learn how to make a transition and remain in a position. Creating an array of perturbations in positions in a safe manner is important, so that the range of disturbances the child can allow and accept grows and develops.

In Figure 4.7, we see the beginning of a transitional movement from sitting to being on the stomach.

The child begins in a sitting position with their knees open, feet wide apart, and the right heel closer to the body than the left. A toy crocodile is in front of the child. The child's attention is drawn into a playful interaction with the crocodile. It is important to observe the lumbar and thoracic curves in the sitting position: the lumbar spine is rounded backward and the curve of the thoracic spine is inward.

As the movement progresses in photos a) to c), these curves of the lumbar and thoracic spine become even more pronounced. As the sequence progresses, the weight of the trunk comes forward over the hip joints with no change in the position of the knees. The head and eyes are focused on the toy, with the head continuously moving and adjusting to the change of position and balance. With the movement of the head, the thoracic curve continues to increase in each of the photos. The lumbar curve changes from being in a flexed, rounded backward position in the top row, to an extended, rounded inward position in photos d) and photo e).

CASE EXAMPLE JANIS—THE KNOWN AS A BASIS FOR THE NEW

When I first met Janis, she could not do any movements on her own. She was able to lie on her back for some time, but would not tolerate being on her side and strongly protested at being put on her stomach. She was able sit upright on the floor with her legs open in front of her, and this was her preferred position. However, she would stiffen in this position and not allow herself to move more than a centimeter in any direction. If moved off her center, Janis could not control any of her movements and would immediately fall in any direction to the floor. Yet in her sitting position, she could stay completely stable.

The process of assisting her to feel movement in the basic directions of forward, backward, and back to the center, and then from left to right and back to the center, required tremendous caution and sensitivity, so as not to arouse any fear or reaction that would cause insecurity. Through my hands and tone of voice, she learned that I would not do anything fast, and that if the degree of being off center was too much or too rapid, that I would immediately stop, return her, and wait for her to regain composure. Once her sense of trust in me and our movements became more stable, it very slowly became possible to create larger movements out of and away from her known and trusted sitting position. Treating this position as a safe haven to move into and away from allowed me to begin to introduce the idea, sensation, and experience of transitioning to somewhere else. It was crucial to find a way to ensure that the initiation of a transition would be experienced as seamless by Janis. Once she had trust in this kind of moving experience, it was possible to enlarge her repertoire in many directions and movements. Each time Janis was introduced to a new and more challenging position and the transition into it, she would become hesitant and insecure. As long as I respected this and went over each small element of the transition in a slow and seamless manner, she would accept, be interested in, and also enjoy the new transitions.

Janis can now be guided toward almost any transition to other positions on her own. She has developed through learning how to increase the range of directions of movement in sitting, and this has given her flexibility in her muscles and joints, which was previously unimaginable. She now enjoys moving and being moved in a variety of ways and being challenged. She can now sense and feel her body and be present while in motion, rather than being in a state of anxiety about what will happen next, wishing to hold onto the only position she knew well. The idea of being able to move and get somewhere on her own is now part of her self-image. She is more communicative, interactive, and responsive. For Janis, learning the intradynamics of sitting became the basis for her to expand the entire understanding of her body in motion, from positions to transitions.

Dynamics of positions and transitions

Regarding the dynamics of positions and transitions, it is important to know and understand that

- positions can be learned and improved in the position itself;
- transitions can be improved during the transition;
- positions can be improved to help transitions, and transitions can be used to help positions;
- the order in which to arrive at and form a developmental position or transition is highly flexible and not predetermined;
- the idea that one phase of development must directly follow another is not practical in therapeutic developmental learning, depending on the age of the child;
- elements of movements or full patterns of motion of later phases can be introduced, used, and learned if patterns and movements of earlier phases are lagging behind, not progressing, or are not fully formed;
- the entire process with special needs children is very malleable with regard to which transition or position can be learned and in which order.

Walking can be learned by walking. It can also be learned by going through the developmental movements that precede it, such as crawling, coming onto one foot and knee, and cruising.

Walking is learned in walking; getting up to standing is learned by doing it. There are many things that can be learned to assist in the learning of walking, but *the functional ability is learned by performing the act itself.*

It might be questioned whether learning a 'more advanced' ability or position before the child has accomplished preceding movements, such as crawling or sitting, will interfere or even harm the new, more advanced ability. An answer is that if all elements to prepare for being more advanced are part of forming new movement ability, it follows that if you are able to accomplish the new ability or function, i.e., be in the position itself, then this must mean that all prior elements will now be incorporated. There is also no logic to thinking that once a more advanced ability is developing you cannot have the child return to a previous functional ability.

Learning is not an all-or-nothing process; you don't need to learn something fully before moving on to the next thing. Each newly learned ability can complement and improve another. If we think that the development of a function/ability/movement/position can or must proceed in a certain way only, then we are not adhering to and practically implementing the biological and evolutionary principle of variation.

4.5 Reversibility and the order of development

Reversibility: The idea of *reversibility* is used in many fields, including psychology, computer science, chemistry, and many more. When applying the idea of reversibility to movement and learning, one interpretation would be that a voluntary movement should be able to go in a specific direction, stop at any point along the line of the movement, and return directly to the beginning along the same line or continue again or stop and change direction, whenever wanted or needed (Feldenkrais, 1972; Hanson, 1958). Reversibility can also be applied when thinking about the development of movement and the learning it requires.

The example of learning to sit: Take the example of a child learning to sit up. One perspective would be that the child needs to know and have experienced many movements that precede sitting up in order to learn how to arrive and remain in a sitting position. In a sense, this says that sitting encompasses all the aspects that came before it. Conversely, it could be said that the child could first learn how to sit and then go in the opposite direction, to learn how to go from sitting back to being on the floor.

It might also be said that the child cannot or will not be able to sit up or 'find their way' to sitting unaided, but could maintain a sitting position if put into it. Using the idea of reversibility, it is possible to develop an earlier developmental ability after having learned a more developed one, or by using elements from a more developed ability to learn a completely different one, provided it contains similar elements.

A question to be asked then is whether the child who cannot sit on their own will experience any benefit from being put into a sitting position and learning how to sit by engaging with the dynamics of sitting in the position itself. Is this of any value for the child's brain and development?

Developmental sequence: A child can learn what is needed for a position or a movement in a variety of other similar situations. Many developmental situations contain aspects of the movement the child needs to learn (Figure 4.8 and Figure 4.9). The order of the movement sequences is not necessarily what helps the aspects of the musculoskeletal patterns to emerge, which are needed to move on to the next developmental movement. It is always possible to return to fill in gaps, i.e., aspects of development that were previously not accomplished fully or even not at all, later on.

This is very much the basis of the work of Dr. Moshe Feldenkrais and his success in working with adults. One of the main ways in which

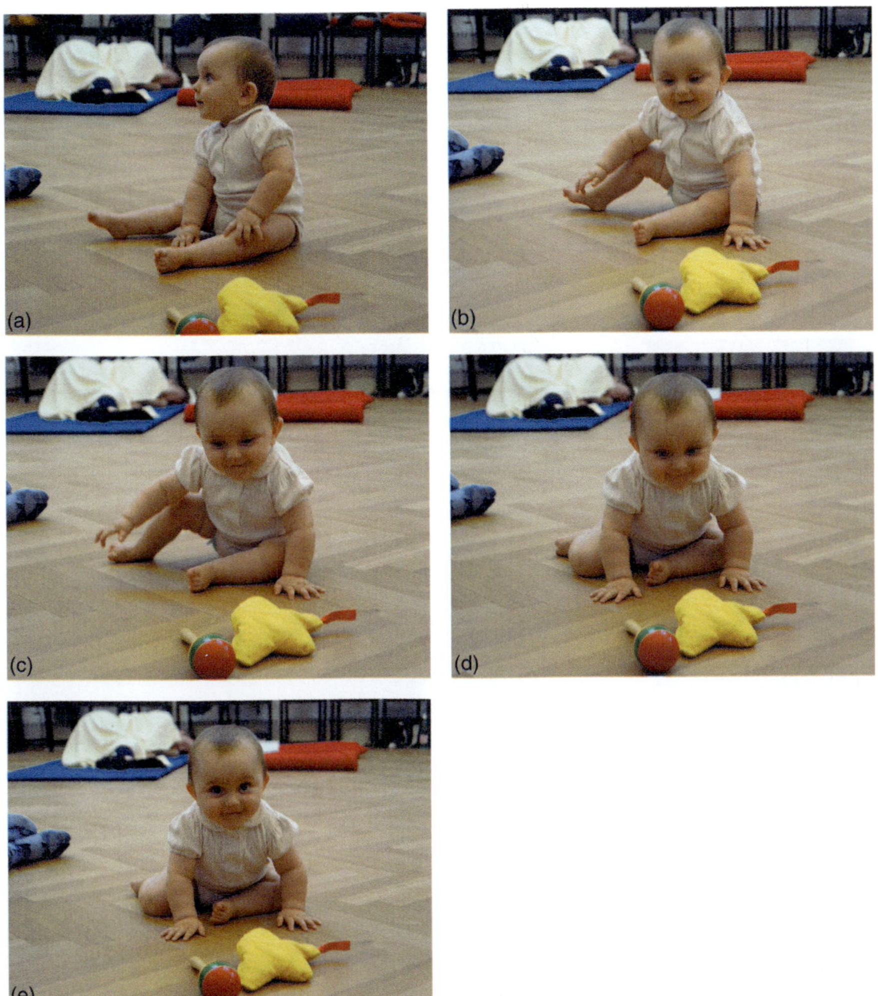

Figure 4.8: Transitional movement 5

Dr. Feldenkrais approached adult leaning was to have people get down onto the floor and lie on their back. While on the floor, they explored and rediscovered movements as adults which they had not learned most efficiently at an earlier age. In essence, this represents revisiting previous or earlier aspects of one's movement that had not been learned in the optimal way for oneself, in order to then return to the upright and perceive, feel, and experience changes and improvements in the upright functions, movements, and experiences.

This fits with the concepts of reversibility, variables of variation, plasticity, and learning.

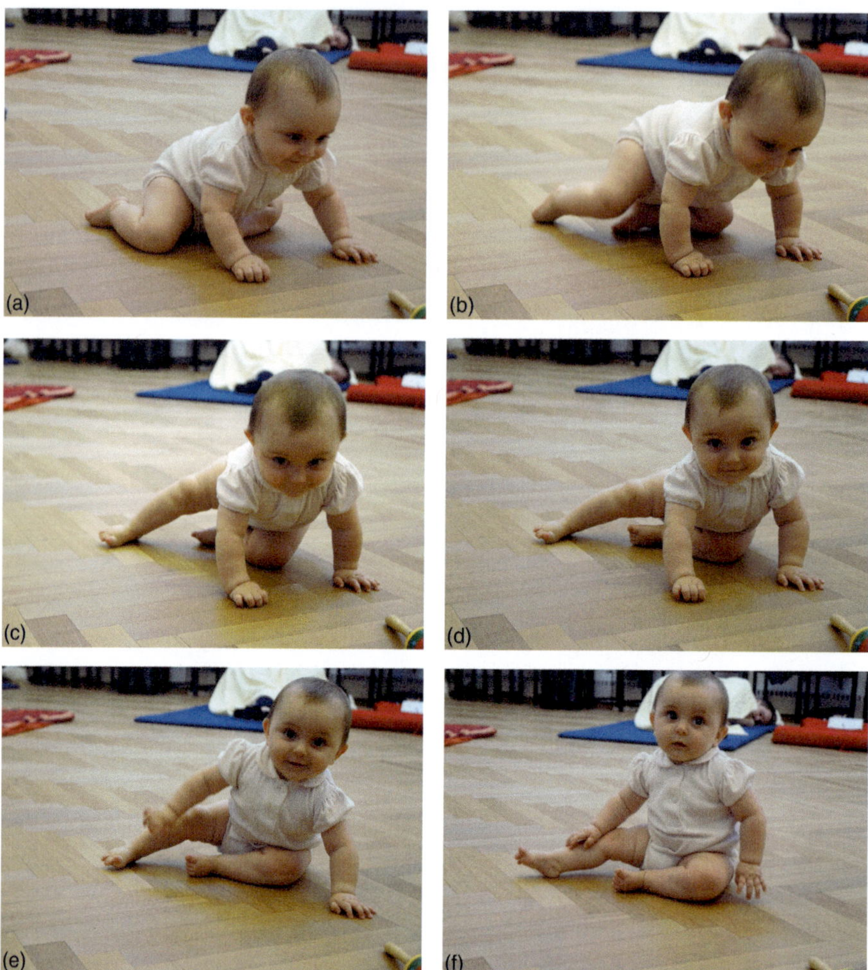

Figure 4.9: Transitional movement 6

The photo sequences in Figure 4.8 and Figure 4.9 illustrate the basic concept of reversibility in developmental movement.

In Figure 4.8, the child starts in an unsupported sitting position and turns 90 degrees around themselves to come to a side-sitting position supported on both hands.

In photo a), the child is sitting with their legs wide outstretched in front of their body and their head in the vertical.

In photo b), the child turns to the left. The distance between the feet remains the same. The left knee bends and the left hand comes to the floor in front of the left hip joint, in line with the left thigh and knee. The head leans forward over the trunk in the direction of the left knee, as the right knee bends and comes off the floor.

In photo c), the weight of the head moves further forward, with the entire trunk leaning over the left thigh via movement in the left hip joint. The right knee turns inward, with the inside of the right foot coming onto the floor.

In photo d), both hands come to the floor to support the weight of the body, as the head is now in front of the left lower leg. The right knee has turned inwards and come down to the floor.

In photo e), the child now sits in a side-sitting position with their head and chest lifted, looking forward with their head and eyes after having completed the turn and transition to the side-sitting position.

In Figure 4.9, the process is reversed, with the child starting in a side-sitting position and ending up in a sitting position without support from their hands. This is a reversal of what takes place in Figure 4.8, where the child starts in a sitting position without support from the hands and ends up in a side-sitting position supported by both hands.

Unique children, unique solutions   5

In order to respect a child's individuality, creativity is required when selecting and trying out the methods available to address the child's particular needs. Every child is unique in terms of the skills and characteristics defining their thinking, communication, and learning behavior. Whether a particular approach is rewarding can be recognized most reliably by its results. However, while results may manifest in obvious change, they may also be more subtle, e.g., alterations in the quality of a movement. Reactions such as mirroring and reinforcing can lend meaning to important progress. Although a child's individual pace must be respected, change and progress should be continuous; if this is not the case, the chosen approach should be reconsidered and a different one selected. A safe environment that conveys security and openness encourages playful activity, which promotes development of motor, situational problem-solving, and attention-control skills. It is important to be prepared for change and progress and to respond to it in a calm but alert manner.

5.1 Strategies for approaching children

Be creative: Each special needs child is unique in terms of their neuromusculoskeletal organization and growth, but also in terms of their unique rhythm of and timeline for developing abilities. General patterns, models, criteria, guiding principles, and parameters can be observed, and certain practices may possibly be followed, as they apply to certain general conditions or diagnoses the child may have. Special needs children are unique in the way they assimilate kinesthetic, sensory, emotional, and

DOI: 10.4324/9781003737988-5

cognitive information and in how they process information for learning and developing their own ways to move and act (Krauss, 1988).

Applying standard practices may sometimes be necessary and successful. The challenge of working with a special needs child's uniqueness is encountered when the standard procedures and practices don't achieve results and improvement. *Unique children require unique solutions.* This requires creative thinking to find ways of presenting the ideas and information the child needs to access. The functional abilities that are needed and important for development are the same for all children—the child's unique way of learning and our approach to accessing this are not. The goal is to find the best way to help a child's abilities emerge, grow, and develop, according to how they learn and not according to how we want to teach.

Frequently, the same tactics and formulas are used over and over again, even if no improvement is seen. When this happens, it is important not to assume that the child can't learn, but rather to reflect on the possibility that it is how we are communicating the teaching or what and how we think the child needs to learn at a given time that is at fault.

Communication and verbal skills: Each special needs child is unique and the spectrum of their communication and verbal abilities is broad. Some children will begin to do a movement only when you guide them through the movement verbally. It may be that you need to verbalize every detail of the movement and describe what is happening moment by moment, for example, where they need to put their elbow, what the pressure will feel like, the rhythm in which they are moving, how far away the floor is, when their foot lifts (Knapp, Hall, & Horgan, 2007). It can be any singular component of the movement or expression of the entire sequence. Sometimes during verbalization of the details of the movement, the tone of your voice needs to be varied, e.g., soft or loud, strong or subtle. This gives the child the necessary cues to connect the interactive touching and the sensory feedback they need. This can aid them in gauging when they need to pay attention and where to focus. It may not matter whether you speak the same language; it is the tone, timing, and rhythm of what you are saying and expressing that are important.

Repetition and variation: Some children benefit from having more pauses and resting periods, and others from constant interaction and information presented over a sustained period of time without a break. Talking to the child in a variety of tones and speeds, singing, humming, whistling, or being quiet during a session are variations that are important to consider.

Changing the order of what is done during each movement or the order of what is done during the session can help certain children. Others need a set order for how they are moved or what movements are presented to them at which point during the learning session. An example of this is the way to sit. Some children will learn sitting or how to come to sitting by doing it in one way only. After this one way has been learned and assimilated, they can tolerate being shown other ways to arrive at sitting or varieties of sitting. Helping a child to understand one situation and only afterwards broadening this to an understanding of novel varieties of the same situation is one approach. In order to be able to assimilate the idea of sitting or of how to come to sitting, another child may need to be presented with a constant variety of ways and positions of sitting and how to come to sitting before the idea of sitting or the idea of coming to sitting is discovered and understood.

The following paragraphs highlight examples of what it means to learn an idea in one specific way or to learn an idea through variations of the idea:

- Ideas in movement can be presented as either a component of the movement or the entire movement. Some children learn to recognize and understand a new movement when one part of the movement is presented to them at a time. In this way, they begin to recognize the movement and sense the parts of themselves that are involved in the particular small element. Once they are familiar with one element of an entire pattern, then they are able to go on to the next.
- When presented element by element in either a sequential or a random order, the child is gradually able to fit the entire sequence together and recognize and develop the ability to perform it. Others need to be offered an entire sequence of a movement fully strung together in order to begin to develop the ability. Only after the whole pattern of motion has emerged and begun to form can they recognize singular elements of the sequence. Both ways are equally important, as elements of one sequence of movement often represent components that can also be used in a different sequence. This is also true for an entire pattern of movement. Different sequences of movement can be put together to form longer ones or used as a variation.
- The ability to transfer the learning arrived at in an interactive therapeutic learning situation is very important. It is often taken for granted or assumed that a child who begins to develop a new movement ability in a therapeutic learning situation will automatically continue with this new skill or ability at home or in other situations. When this does not happen, it may be felt that it was just by chance that a new ability 'showed up' in the interactive learning sessions, or that it 'only' happens with the therapist. This may indeed be the case, but being able to transfer the learning to other situations often requires particular details that are present in the

interactive learning environment but not at home or in other environments. It can be as simple as having the same toys with the same colors, or the same mats, lighting, or music. Taking these particulars into consideration can sometimes be what truly makes a difference. It can help the learning to take hold faster and more effectively.

5.2 Creating a safe environment for playing and learning

Safe surroundings: Feeling safe in the environment you are in is a condition that everyone needs—be they child or adult, young or old. We can only be open and thrive in all aspects of our ourselves when the feeling and sensation of safety are present (Siegel, 2007; Van der Kolk, 2012; Bowlby, 1969; Cozolino, 2006; De Waal, 2009).

An environment that gives the child a feeling of safety and openness is an environment where the child feels secure and confident enough to play. Play for typically developing children is the usual state and is spontaneous. When entering a new environment, a child who has reached the age where they have begun to play will quickly look for objects to play with. However, they will only do this when they feel secure and confident in the situation and surroundings (Figure 5.1). They will occupy themselves with a toy, explore the room, and engage with others.

Ability development through play: Engaging in playful activity is a biological imperative for the young, as can be seen in many species of the animal world. Play is very important for the developing brain. It is driven and motivated by curiosity and interest in the objects and people in the immediate environment. Children play by themselves, with their parents and siblings, and after a period of time, they learn to play with other children. The activity of playing involves creativity, imagination, exploration, adventure, new experiences, challenge, and social engagement. Children can develop confidence in themselves through different kinds of play. They develop imagination and play through fantasy while creating complex fictional situations. All of these are used when seeking solutions to more and more complex functional movement situations.

It is very important for the development of the young child's brain to learn with and through play. An environment that encourages self-play as well as interactive play is one in which the child has confidence and feels secure and safe. Positive human relationships are the building blocks of healthy development. Play can be used to develop motor abilities, situational problem-solving, and attention-focusing skills.

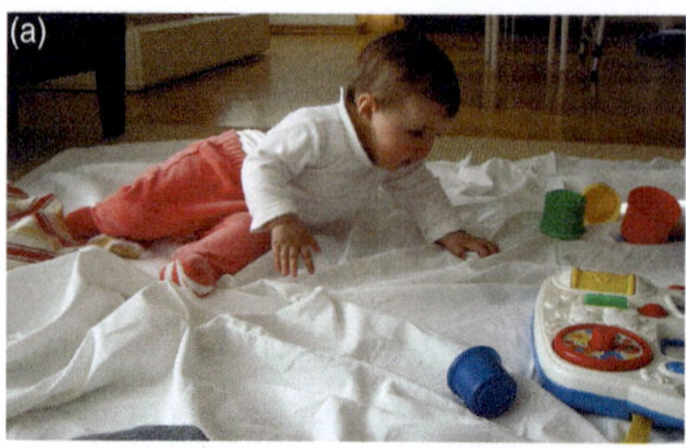
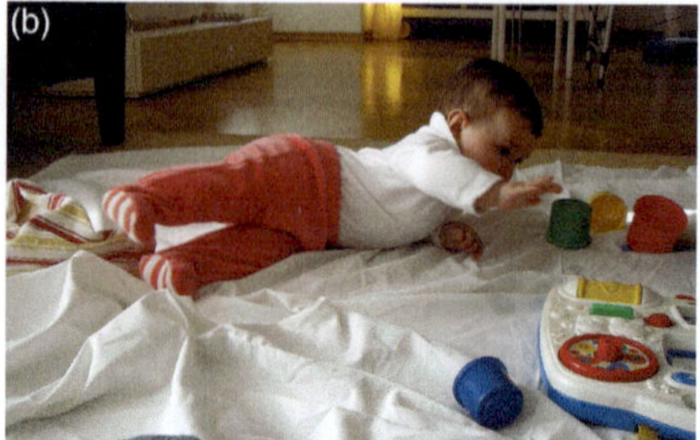
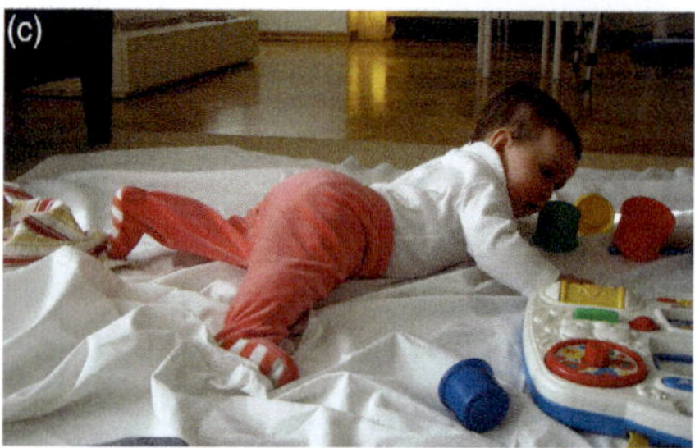

Figure 5.1: Playful exploration and discovery

In Figure 5.1, we see a fully engaged and interested child surrounded by toys, in a safe place on the floor to explore and play.

In photo a), the child is supporting itself on their left hand. The chest and upper back are turned around the left shoulder joint, and the left arm is in front of the head and chest. The left leg is bent on the floor in front, and the right leg is bent behind. The chest has no contact with the floor.

In b), the child begins to reach toward something on the floor that has attracted their attention and focus. The child lowers themself onto the left forearm and elbow. Both legs straighten with the feet flexed. The right leg is in the air. The child's back is extended, with the chest hanging forward to the floor and the right side bent.

In photo c), the child arrives with their right hand on the floor. The extension of the back and the side-bending are maintained; the head remains in the air. The right leg comes forward to the floor, and the left leg is somewhat bent, in line with the left side of the body. The head and eyes remain focused on the object of interest. The belly comes into contact with the floor.

Establish contact: One of the initial goals with a special needs child is to find a way to come into good contact with them. This requires synchronizing with the child and developing an in-sync relationship. An in-sync relationship is one where the child feels you do things and engage together, match each other, and interact via movement with or without touch, both verbally and nonverbally. With this type of relationship and interaction, the child feels interpersonally that they are accepted; they trust the entire situation, so that play is possible, accepted, and allowed. With many special needs children, achieving this state is not an easy task, yet the time and effort spent arriving in such a state are well worth it. There is no one way to do this. Each special needs child is different in terms of their early experiences and sensory-emotional processing. This is something that can be taught and learned with very clear and practical processes.

The first step is learning how to be present and attentive to specific cues from the child as well as to one's own responses to these cues.

5.3   How can change be gauged?

The appropriateness of what is done is determined by the results and improvements that are achieved. Knowing which strategy and methodology to choose is challenging. One must be attentive and mindful in order to recognize when the applied approach is not working, and not wait too long before attempting something different. One of the biggest errors you can make is to think that what you are doing would work, but that the child cannot grasp it.

Evaluation of responses and results: Watching for the child's response and knowing what to look for in that response is essential. It can be seen rather quickly whether what is being attempted with the child is accomplishing that which they set out to do. Once this is clear, it is then possible to either continue until the goal is achieved or to change strategy, review the thinking, and try something new. Many children try many different therapies and methods if they don't find the solutions they are searching for. Searching for unique solutions to unique, seemingly unsolvable problems is a continuous challenge. Finding new ways to help children requires determination and resolve. It requires unwavering belief in the human spirit and the incomparable courage that these children show in the face of the challenges they live with day in and day out.

Observe progress: To observe and sense progress in the developmental abilities of a child, one must be able to see and sense with one's hands when change happens, where it has changed, and what has changed. Some people have set preconceptions and ideas of what it means to have something change in a developmental ability.

Among these preconceptions is that for change to happen, it must be something 'very big' or 'very significant,' and that only certain types of alterations are to be considered 'real change' (Hüther, 2006, 2018; Schore, 2012; Stern, 2004). Others may have the thinking that when the final result of an action or movement appears, such as rolling up to sitting or a child that is up and walking, that then—and only then—has change and progress taken place. The viewpoint is that anything less is 'not real change or progress.'

There is a wide spectrum of significant changes that can take place in developmental abilities. Changes can be big or small, subjective or objective, external and/or internal, quantitative or qualitative; there may be shifts in flexibility and tone. Modifications and adjustments of certain variations of particular movements or reactions to the environment and context of the movement are also significant and fall into the domain of 'changes in an ability.'

Visible changes: Changes that are external are easier to observe and explain to others. External changes may also be large or small. The larger the change in a movement ability, the easier it is to point out to another person. When the change is small, it may seem insignificant and not noticeable.

Parents of typically developing very young infants often notice the smallest of changes that take place from day to day. When the changes in the movements are larger, there is less of a tendency to observe and notice them, unless they are as significant as the change from one phase to another, such as from not crawling to crawling, sitting up, coming up to standing, and taking the first steps. For the special needs child, all changes are important, and all need to be given observational significance. Any change—small or large—in the direction of developmental formation takes on great significance. Each and every new change signifies that change and growth of new functions *is* taking place and continuously reinforces that abilities are being learned and growing. Every change can be built upon to help generate the emergence of a new ability and foster further development of neural movement networks.

Understanding how to notice and sense change is a skill that is needed to help others, such as parents or other professionals, make sense of the progressive developmental changes that take place in a special needs child. Being able to clearly point out and explain the specifics of whatever changes take place in any domain helps others to 'see' the particular child and the progress they are making more clearly. It assists in helping others focus on specific changes.

Invisible changes: Changes that are internal and subjective are not easily noticed by an untrained observer. An example of this is the sensation of change in the quality of a movement. It may be that the movement is perceived to be smoother, easier, require less effort, or flow better. Another example is the perception of the sensation of the movement itself. Some children do not have clear sensations of a movement when it is being performed. This is often the case with special needs children. When a movement has never been done before and is experienced for the first time, it may be difficult for the child to perceive the new sensation. When the child is asked to follow or carry out the movement by themself and the sensation of the movement is unclear, it may be difficult and awkward to do. After a number of repetitions, the sensation, sequence, and pattern of the movement may become more present, available, and clearer to perceive.

CASE EXAMPLE JULIE—SMALL CHANGES, BIG PROGRESS

Julie was a sweet child of 3 years with a very rare genetic deletion. Her face was mostly without expression, and she struggled to focus her eyes for any length of time. When she did manage to focus, it was not clear whether she was focusing on someone or something, or just staring into space. Although she was 3 years old, Julie was not able to perform early developmental movements, such as rolling from her back to her side and onto her stomach, and could not find her way to sitting or push up onto her knees. She also could not hold herself up when placed in a sitting position, nor could she support her head in any direction. If put in a sitting position, she would immediately collapse and fall forward unless supported completely. Thus, when put in a sitting position, Julie needed supports behind her to lean her head against; if her head was brought forward, it would immediately drop and hang down.

There was much work to be done to find a direction of movement in which to proceed to enable Julie to make progress and possibly begin to hold her head. First, a means had to be found to enable Julie to feel, sense, and move any part of her body from one position to another, and maintain it for even the shortest time.

It was also not known whether Julie could comprehend what was said to her, or whether she could locate the parts of her body sensory-wise and possibly control them movement-wise. When interacting with children, I speak, talk, and sing to them a lot. The children I see come from all over the world, with many different mother tongues, and singing and/or talking has a potent and profound effect on all of them. This is an essential form of communication, since the voice is a tool to make and maintain contact, as well as with which to express and convey emotion, sensation, direction, and the various forms of movement interaction. It is important to use varieties of intonations and rhythms of the voice to reach a child, whatever aspect of learning is required and sought.

At the beginning of working with Julie, it seemed important to talk to her, even though there was no indication that she could comprehend or make sense of voice or intonation or even knew that someone was speaking to her. As the relationship with Julie grew, using voice and speaking to her began to take on an increasingly central role. Verbalizing the specific movements that were being learned through hands-on guidance as well as where each body part would go or not go became a continuous conversation of communication and monitoring.

One day during a session, Julie was boosted up to sitting by leaning against some mats which are firm enough to give support but soft enough to protect in the event of a fall, with her head leaning backward onto the mat behind. From this position, I began to very carefully bring her forward in a central direction, so that the head would have to be lifted slightly to continue coming forward and not fall backward onto the mat. With a rather demanding firm voice, I said, 'Julie, keep your head up!' There seemed to be a very noticeable and clear split-second response in which Julie held her head. It was a special moment to be present at and observe, as it seemed that she did comprehend, could follow, and respond to what was said to and asked of her. But the response was so small as to beg the question, 'Did she really just do that or was it just chance?' Her mother was very attentive to any small or large changes she saw, and it seemed that she had also picked up on it. The next two or three repetitions yielded no response, but then, on the fifth attempt, it was there again just as clearly.

When working with children like Julie, repetition of a response will not be seen each and every time, sometimes not even on the same day. For an ability to begin to emerge, it just needs to happen more than once in any timeframe and then begin to happen more and more often. With Julie, the response to a demanding voice and the specific direction asked of her began to appear clearly and repeatedly, observable to all present during the sessions. Either Julie understood from the tonality or rhythm of the voice or the words spoken, or both.

Sometime later it became apparent that repeating the specific direction of movement very quickly or loudly, or with different tonalities at different points in the movement, made a very big difference to the rate of response and the direction of the movement. Julie began to bring her head back to the middle from almost any position off center when it was asked of her. She was able to stay stable for longer with her head upright, centered, and stable. Her eyes started to focus more often and for longer periods of time. She began to initiate and make eye contact, and, after a while, began to smile and show a greater variety of emotional expression. This continued to happen on a steady basis and not haphazardly. The abilities were no longer in the emergent but now in the developing stage.

It was fascinating to watch how Julie's ability to follow and control her movements grew and grew, along with a new and varied repertoire of using her new, developing abilities. It took months of diligent work for Julie to fully bring up her head and keep it up in various positions, from being on her back and coming up to sitting, to being on her hands and knees, and even up to standing. Julie is now able to focus her eyes, make clear and steady contact with other people, and take steps and walk with assistance. Julie's entire process of progress started with one very briefly observed moment that could easily have been missed, not paid attention to or not awarded any significance.

Individual pace and continuity: While working with Julie, it was essential not to have a finger on a stopwatch or a calendar, but rather to work with Julie's individual and consistent rate of improvement and progress. The timeline was defined by each and every new element that emerged, which showed itself as Julie's unique rate of learning. One has to see change, progress, and development to be able to adjust and find the developmental timeline of each special needs child.

Even among typically developing children, the rhythms and timelines vary enormously regarding how and when a child reaches and develops each new phase of ability development—phases which eventually culminate in standing, walking, and speaking.

The quintessential point is that there must be a *continuum of progress in the developmental direction*. Once progress is clearly observed, then the realistic expectations of the rhythm and timeline of development are easier to understand and accept.

Experience change: For a special needs child, a movement is often very difficult to perform, and the sensation is clouded by the difficulty. When there is a change in the ease of the movement done by or to the child, the sensation will be less clouded, and the perception of the sensation of the movement itself will become easier to distinguish (Feldenkrais, 1972, 1981). These changes are important for the child but not easily observed from the outside. For a child, experiencing these kinds of changes together with another person who acknowledges and responds to them lends the experience of change significance and meaning. The internal relevance of a new experience involving change is rooted in the emotional as well as in the kinesthetic world of the child. When there is meaning, it becomes easier for the child to remember these new changes in their movement abilities and makes it easier to apply them. It gives priority and importance to sensations that would otherwise not be paid attention to or focused on. A skill set needs to be developed that enables one to sense and feel changes in the ease, quality, and perception of the variety of changes that are possible. For this, it is very important and useful to learn how to create such changes in oneself.

Giving meaning to change: It is important to know how to give significance and meaning to a change that takes place in a child. Many special needs children are nonverbal and may also be cognitively challenged. Emotions, sensations, and new movements; responses to changes; and new adaptations to situations do not necessarily have meaning for the child (Knapp, Hall, & Horgan, 2007). One way in which infants and toddlers learn how to give and assign meaning to any aspect of a situation is by experiencing this together with another person (Schore, 1994; Krauss, 1988; Frankl, 1959).

A child does not know whether something is significant or not. Sharing of the moment creates an opportunity to point out significance and, in doing so, give it meaning. This can be achieved by the tone of voice, a particular sound, an expression, a change in the force of the grip on the child, a change in speed, a repetition, or a reinforcement. It can be done through encouragement as well as by discouragement. As long as the child can be attentive to the fact that 'what is happening now is something different' and can internally mark that this is important, it can promote growth and development. If it is emphasized and pointed out in some way, then there is a greater chance that the child will give it meaning. The clearer the meaning, the greater the possibility that the child will retain the significance of the experience and store it as a memory. This memory can have one, two, many, or all of the components of the moment. The more components it retains, the higher the possibility that the changes will develop into long-term changes.

Observing change in oneself: This is the value for adults, parents, and therapists of having experience in self-learning through movement, such as gleaned in the JKA Abilities Lessons in Movement. Self-learning takes on importance for helping to create, recognize, and assign meaning to something that is changing. If, as an adult, we can become more attuned and sensitive to changes in our bodies and Self and also recognize their significance, these experiences become a practical and important skill when present together with a child as change emerges. Once the internal mechanics of change are learned in oneself, it becomes easier to sense these types of changes when working with a child. This is the value of adult self-experiential learning through movement. The learned skills of self-observation of change can then be transferred to working hands-on with children and adults. These are important skills to learn, because all changes need to be verbalized and explained to a parent or another professional.

5.4   Expecting the unexpected—being ready, mindful, and present

Be prepared: One must train oneself to understand and view dynamic movement situations with thinking and preparedness. What a special needs child does, will do, or could do in the next moment should never come as a surprise. This means being prepared with your hands, thinking, and within your own movement organization, so that you can imagine the variety of options in any movement situation that is being explored or developed by and with the child. One must always be prepared to act with the child in whatever movement may come next, or to lead it from the present movement into the next (Siegel, 2007).

React to the unexpected: *Dynamic thinking and movement interaction* with a child enable one to be present in the moment. They permit an uninterrupted flow of the feelings and sensations of movement, both for the child and for oneself. The sensation for the child is that there are no corners, edges, hesitancies, or breaks in the stream of movement progression they are learning or which is occurring spontaneously via the movement interaction. It demands concentrated attention, vigilance, and constant readiness to adapt to the unexpected. At the same time, it requires a sensitive and well-cultivated internal understanding and personal experience of the subtleties of the movements themselves. This, in turn, predisposes a process of first studying and learning how this pertains to a typically developing child, and then applying the practical knowledge to a special needs child.

Know variations and combinations: The distinct movement transitions and positions seen in a typically developing baby during all the developmental phases of the first 18 months of life can be categorized and studied.

However, the number of possible combinations and variations of these dynamic transitional movements is immense, and they would be very difficult to categorize exactly. How each individual child alters, varies, adapts, reacts, and responds to both the social and physical environment through their movements is not easy to predict and follow. This is because the situations themselves are dynamic and embedded within a specific context in each and every distinct moment. One time, the child may react to a situation and move in one way, and the next time they may react very differently. It is thus essential to be prepared and able to anticipate the next direction in which the child may move.

It is important to know not only the transitions, positions, and diversity of combinations and variations, but also to try out and explore different kinds of transitions, positions, combinations, and variations of movement oneself. This takes on even greater significance when working with special needs children, with their highly unique ways of moving and responding.

Don't be surprised: The diversity of muscular organization, skeletal structures, and tonal differences is enormous among special needs children. The types of asymmetries in a child's movements due to different muscular physiology and their effect on skeletal growth in each of the limbs vary hugely. Particularities of the way the child moves because of these factors mean that it is not easy to know 'what's next.' Some children move suddenly with great speed and force from one movement to another. Other children have had surgery or wear ankle foot orthoses (AFOs) and need them on during the session. Some may be standing with good tone and then, in less than a second, buckle at the knees, lose all tone, and become like a rag doll. All of these factors need to be taken into consideration when thinking about 'not being surprised' by the direction, speed, or force of the child's movement.

It takes training and experience to become proficient in knowing and reacting spontaneously and fluidly to the different possible movements a child can present at any given moment. For over 40 years, I have trained myself to never be surprised by a child's next movement. This is one of the most important factors to know and one of the essential skills to have acquired when starting to work with a child. It is a skill set that can be learned, studied, and practiced. How quickly and smoothly you can move with any child, no matter how and in which direction they move 'all of a sudden' or 'in a split second,' is of vital importance. This pertains not only to the movement itself, but also to the responses and reactions of the child and yourself during the dynamic movement interaction with the child.

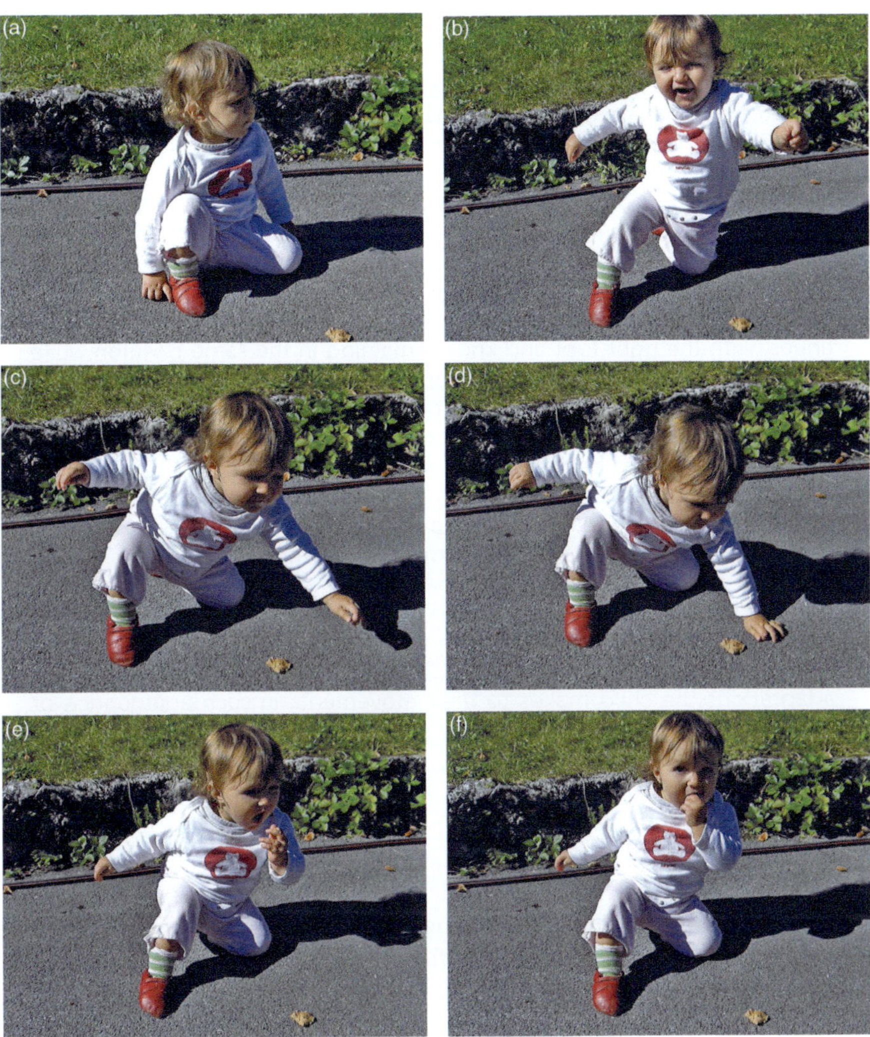

Figure 5.2: Understanding dynamic movement situations

In the photo sequence shown in Figure 5.2, we see a child move through a number of unstable positions on one knee and foot. The child needs to be able to coordinate and adapt to the unstable changes that take place during the movement.

In photo a), the child is in a sitting position on the ground with their right knee placed directly over their foot. The arms hang at the sides of the body.

In photo b), the child comes directly up onto the left knee while the right knee maintains its position over the right foot. As this takes place, the arms lift, one arm moving forward and one arm backward. The forearm and shoulder joint of each arm rotate in a slightly different direction as the child's head comes into the vertical, looking forward.

In c), the left hip flexes and the pelvis goes backward and to the right as the left arm goes down toward the floor. The movement of the trunk is free and without hesitation, hinging over both hip joints. The right knee and foot are stable as the knee maintains its position over the foot.

In photo d), the hinging movement of the trunk at the hip joints continues, with the right foot and knee remaining in the same position while the left hand comes down to the ground.

In photo e), the left hand lifts from the floor and the right knee and lower leg move a bit further inward to the left. The trunk lifts, and with it the right arm moves backward and down, while the left side of the pelvis goes farther backward.

In f), the child's head returns to the vertical and the right knee returns to being over the foot, where it has remained in every photo except e). The right arm continues to turn and go backward.

Placing one's hands on the child's pelvis from behind, to follow the movements without interfering, one would have to be very fluid in one's own movements; be ready, mindful, and present for all the changes and adaptations the child makes to their movements in such a sequence or another of a similar nature.

5.5   Moments of experience

The moments of experience a child encounters during a therapeutic learning session are diverse and of great significance for the child. They must not be passed over as though meaningless or secondary. To be present, mindful, and attentive to a child's moment of experience is one of the foundations of a developmental movement interaction (Stern, 2004).

Moments of experience occur while the child is simultaneously occupied by a dynamic interface of learning new movements and developing new skills. A few of these moments are listed below:

- moments of wonder, amazement, joyfulness, and laughter;
- moments of success, pride, and self-confidence;
- moments of curiosity, attention, and self-discovery;
- moments of figuring it out;
- moments of going somewhere;
- moments of motivation and interest;

- moments of staying still;
- moments of needing assistance;
- moments of uncertainty, confusion, and fear of the unknown;
- moments of frustration, challenge, and difficulty;
- moments of failure.

Paying attention to these special moments lends an added facet to the child's experience. It allows them to feel that they are sharing these moments with someone, that they are not alone in what is happening. The shared experience adds further depth and dimension to the movements and abilities that are emerging and developing. All experiences that interconnect with the developing movements create a richness in the neural networking and intertwine into a collective neuromuscular, emotional, and sensory pattern. The broader and more varied the experiences, the greater the chance that they will grow from short-term into longer-term memories—memories of both the experience itself and the movements learned at the time.

The short- and long-term goal is to give the child wide-ranging moments of experience. These will include positive as well as more difficult and challenging moments, all of which are part of the life experience. Developing a greater tolerance of both positive and challenging sensory-emotional movement experiences gives the child the strength and confidence they need to continue learning and growing. This pertains not only to the special needs of the child in motion, but also to the special needs of the child as a person who faces unique challenges in life as they develop and grow. Respecting their individual moments of experience is impactful, a great contribution that one can make and a gift to the child.

The considerable variety of moments of experience, each with its own qualities and characteristics, accounts for a wide spectrum of the human condition in life. Being present in moments of experience can be transformative for the child.

Moments of wonder, amazement, joyfulness, and laughter: These can occur when the unexpected happens for the child and, all of a sudden, the child finds themselves in a new position or accomplishing a movement they have never done before or never thought they would.

Being joyful with a child or sharing laughter is a powerful moment to experience. A child can become joyful or laugh very suddenly and spontaneously. During an interactive situation, when your thinking and focus are elsewhere, the child may show wonder and joyfulness and begin to laugh! Sharing this moment with the child helps to heighten the experience.

Shifting focus from what you are occupied with and focused on, so that your state of experience is the same as that of the child, lends greater significance to the moment.

Moments of success, pride, and self-confidence: Any time a child accomplishes something new—or arrives in a situation they have been trying to master for some time and finally do—can be a moment of pride for the child. When the child struggles with something but does not give up on themselves, the moment they arrive at doing it can be a moment of success and self-confidence.

Moments of curiosity, attention, and self-discovery: A moment of self-discovery can be when a child suddenly discovers a part of their body, something as seemingly innocent as the discovery of their fingers or toes. Many special needs children have never interlaced their own fingers and seen their own hands and fingers while doing so. They may have never turned the palm of their hand, opened their fingers, and touched and caressed their own face or that of their mother or father. Some have never touched their own feet or toes, or brought their foot close to their mouth, looked at it, then put the toes into their mouth. Others have never crawled or stood up. Moments of self-discovery can be preceded by great moments of curiosity and attention. Some part of the child or some movement they are doing by chance comes into their attention in such a way that they can focus on it. This stirs a moment of curiosity in the child that holds their attention. It is essential to be aware of these distinct moments of curiosity and attention and not to interfere with them. It is possible to heighten these moments by waiting actively with the child and being present with them in their experience of self-discovery.

Moments of figuring (it) out: This happens when some movement or way of doing something—like a child grabbing a toy with their hand by figuring out how to turn the forearm and wrist to allow the fingers to open, so that when they reach to grab a toy the hand is positioned correctly—is discovered. Or perhaps they can already grab a toy but have now figured out how to open the fingers to let it go again. Both are very different functional actions that certain children struggle with. Other examples could be that when rolling up to sitting, the child figures out where to place a hand on the floor to support themselves as they come up, or discovers how they need to shift their weight to be able to lift a foot off the ground to take a step. Moments of figuring out are very special for a child, as they are also moments of self-accomplishment.

Moments of going somewhere: All actions need to start somewhere. A starting position is left to go to and arrive at another. These are moments of going somewhere. When you go somewhere together with someone, you either accompany them or you join in to experience a moment of going somewhere together. The knowledge that you are going somewhere and that you have moved there from another place requires cognition of where you are in space and that another place you go to is different.

There are children who cannot easily make distinctions between one place and another. They may also be hesitant to go somewhere else, particularly if it is somewhere they don't know or can't move to smoothly. A moment of going somewhere can help the child to recognize that they are now transitioning. When you give the child your attention in a way that tells them you understand that they are in a movement moment, then you share this moment with them.

Motivation and interest: These are qualities we take for granted as being part of a child. Children are interested in so many things. They are motivated to move and do and try out whatever they can. They are fascinated by new things and interested in the world around them. However, if you do not recognize what an object is, or you can't use your hand or arm to reach out to it or crawl to move toward it, then you may not have an interest in it or be motivated to want to have it. Watching motivation and interest emerge in a child is precious. Perhaps the child was not interested or motivated just a moment beforehand. When these moments of motivation and interest arrive, we may only witness them—we may not interfere. They are very important moments that can radically change the direction of a child's development. It is very difficult to push a child to be motivated or interested when the ability does not exist. Once it begins to emerge and happen more frequently, we can assume there has been a significant change in the child's brain. As the child develops more moments of interest, it is almost certain that many more new directions will appear in their growth and learning. There is no way to force this aspect of development; each of these moments of motivation and interest must be noted and appreciated.

A moment of staying still: Some children have challenges in staying still. There are neuromuscular conditions that make it very difficult for the child to control their movements, meaning that they can never just stay still. The experience of staying still is unusual, if indeed it occurs at all (possibly only during sleep). A moment of staying still is then a very special moment. There are ways to interact in movement so that the child comes to be still. When they are still, they can also be very quiet and attentive to their surroundings.

In this moment of staying still, it may be that the child's visual perception of who and what they see is different. To be with the child in this quiet and still moment, and to acknowledge the moment by becoming still and quiet in the stillness as well, is what the child needs. It helps them to recognize more clearly the sensation of the moment and the feeling of themself in the stillness.

Moments of needing assistance: Such moments can either promote independence in a child or further a feeling of helplessness in them. It strongly depends on how you behave and interact with the child at the moment of their needing the particular assistance. These are moments that take place during a developmental movement interaction. They can happen so quickly that an outside observer may not even notice. A very short and quick moment, e.g., when, during an interaction, the child is coming from their back by way of their side up to sitting. The smallest moment—when the arm must bend at the elbow, and the head must come far enough forward and over the center of the body so that the child can lean on the elbow and forearm—any small aspect of the movement can pose a challenge for the child. The head may not come forward far enough to shift the weight of the trunk onto the side to cause a clear bending of the body, which allows the elbow to bend. It may be that the forearm needs to turn so that the palm of the hand comes to the floor, or that the elbow itself does not bend smoothly. These elements, and possibly others, may represent the difference between a child being able to do the movement fully and needing a moment of assistance.

Many of these moments are not obvious to an outside observer but are sensed in the interaction itself. They are moments that can fill in and complete a missing component of an entire pattern of motion for the child. Needing assistance and accepting it comes from a feeling of trust in those around us, who we know will lend support no matter what and when. Needing assistance does not make a child smaller but allows them to be vulnerable and well-connected, and have a positive dependence. The more positive experiences they have with others when in need of assistance, the more their ability to use the assistance and not shy away from it or feel it is a sign of weakness and inability will grow. A child who is active in their learning and growth welcomes the challenges that arise. This child is open to all those helping and allows themself to have *moments of needing assistance*.

The child knows that these are not crutches to lean on, but bridges to walk over and use. Attentively observing how the child behaves in these moments of needing assistance is crucial. Extending assistance when it is not needed can further a feeling of helplessness and inability in the child, rather than promoting a positive moment. There is a fine line between denying the child assistance while trying to impose our thinking that they 'need to do it on their own' and observing the child actively and letting them find for themself the moments of needing assistance—in which we must be there and be ready to extend our support at precisely the right moment.

Moments of uncertainty, of confusion, of fear of the unknown: These may arise when the child begins to do a movement and is not sure what comes next or where it is possible to move to, or when the child wants to go further in a particular direction but does not know where it leads or how to return. Uncertainty and confusion also arise when the child becomes disoriented in space or moves in a new direction that they thought would be easy but, all of a sudden, isn't.

Knowing where one is in space is a basic functional requirement of orienting to our immediate surroundings. Our original orientation is toward our mother or primary caregiver. Knowing where they are gives us the knowledge of where we are. There is also orientation toward the space around us in six basic directions: up–down, forward–backward, left–right. These orientations combine and vary when we move in different ways and in different kinds of terrain. Not being able to move in all of these directions limits us.

Everyone has experienced a loss of orientation at one time or another. It can be a very unsettling experience. As an adult, it can happen when waking up suddenly from a deep sleep, or when being disturbed by either something external or something internal, like a nightmare. When we wake up very suddenly and jump up to sit on the bed or stand, we don't know where we are, and we cannot move. We first have to remember where we are, which room we are in, where the door is, how to move, and where to move to. Until we regain clarity, we cannot move anywhere.

Children can also lose their orientation in different ways. In the case of special needs children, they may have never developed a sense of orientation in certain directions and movements.

CASE EXAMPLE JULIAN—'I DID IT!'

Julian was one such child that only had difficulty moving in a certain direction. He was a wonderful young boy with cerebral palsy and a very positive, enthusiastic attitude. He was very motivated to learn, socially outgoing, communicative, and cooperative. Julian was very accepting of every position and direction of movement that needed further learning, except lying down on his back. He simply refused to lie on his back. Any time an attempt to distract or interact with him and head in any direction toward his back was made, even hinted at, Julian would immediately—very stubbornly and with strength—move in another direction.

At first, it seemed that it would pass, and he would easily learn to be on his back. However, as time went on, it became very clear that this was not a simple issue for Julian. Any movement that would bring him in the direction of lying on his back would immediately evoke a strong avoidance response. At even the slightest insistence that he try to lie down on his back, strong signs of panic would ensue. The directions of up, down, right, and left are all within our visual field. We can look up, down, right, and left as we are moving in these directions. All of these directions were fine for Julian, even though it was not clear how good his perception of depth and distance actually was. He could easily go from his side to lying on his stomach or from sitting to standing and was able to maintain his orientation and track where he was going in a smooth controlled manner. Julian certainly had many challenges besides the issue of lying on his back, but when dealing with these, he remained open and happy to learn. This was certainly not the case for his willingness to lie on his back. He had developed many good strategies for avoiding the direction of backward and onto his back.

Going backward is the most challenging and unknown direction to learn. We don't know what is behind us, how far it is to go, and have no way to judge the distance if we cannot see it. It is the last direction that the head learns to move in during early developmental stages. Only when the head is able to stabilize and control itself, so that it does not bang itself when going backward from sitting, does the direction become possible and fluid.

During a session, as he was attending to a toy, Julian misplaced his hand and started to roll backward in the direction of lying on his back. He had momentum and could not stop. His eyes immediately closed and, as a result, all orientation was lost. As this happened, Julian became very huddled up and started to cry heartbreakingly. He did not open his eyes for a number of seconds. It took Julian some time to regain his orientation and know where he was and who he was with, to return to feeling safe in the room and with himself. He needed a lot of comforting and reassurance that everything was okay again. Once the episode was over, he quickly returned to his happy, playful self. Julian would immediately lose his orientation when going backward, which is why he avoided this direction of movement so completely.

A slow and incremental learning sequence would have to be constructed to help Julian learn to keep his orientation while going backward and not become overwhelmed by fear of the unknown. The movement components would have to be small enough for Julian to follow easily without evoking any uncertainty, confusion, and loss of orientation. In this way, he would be able to discover which specific components began to spark the unpleasant response and, in turn, gain control over his reactions so that the fear and anxiety would dissipate.

Julian's first reaction was to close his eyes. We decided to learn together how to maintain constant eye contact and talk to each other while doing movements. This worked well. The next reaction was that he would stiffen his chest and hold his breath. To approach this, Julian needed to learn more about breathing itself. What it feels like to hold your breath and then start breathing again, and how this is connected to stiffening the chest, was a good starting point. Julian became fascinated by different ways of being attentive to himself while in motion. After we had clarified a number of other components of the movement for him, it was time to try to begin with small movements in the direction going onto his back.

Close verbal and visual contact the entire time, and for Julian to know that I was 'right with him' at every moment, was essential. There was the assurance that nothing would be done quickly or as a surprise to him. Any time the slightest sensation of fear or anxiety began to appear, I would raise my voice somewhat and make sure Julian kept his eyes looking directly into mine and did not hold his breath. Once these aspects were under his control, he would no longer lose his orientation in terms of the location of the ceiling, the floor, or any other part of the surroundings. While he was going backward, Julian also needed to keep his attention on the sensation of the surfaces that surrounded him and upon which he was sitting or lying, such as the floor or a table or chair. This was achieved through an exercise of sensing the parts of himself that were in contact with the surface he was lying on. The sensation of the hard surface—and knowing that he was safe on it and in the room—had a very positive impact on him. During this learning process, Julian had moments of success as well as moments of uncertainty, of confusion, and of fear of the unknown. When he succeeded in arriving on his back—with the sensation of the table beneath his body and looking at the ceiling above with calm breathing—there were moments of great pride, stillness, and wonder. There was a particular time when he accidentally fell onto his back without being aware that it was happening. It was an extraordinary moment: Julian looked directly up to the ceiling and then recognized where he was. At the moment of this realization, Julian began to laugh with great joy, saying repeatedly, 'I am on my back! I am on my back! I did it!' Whoever was in the room during all the varied moments of Julian's sessions could not help but be taken in by how he managed his challenges and shared with him this moment of success and pride.

Moments of frustration, challenge, and difficulty: All children experience moments of frustration, challenge, and difficulty—all the more so when the child has special needs. These particular moments are often experienced by the child when they are on the cusp of achieving new developmental progress or a breakthrough into a new phase of development, such as crawling or standing up for the very first time. They may have learned and assimilated all they need to take the next step, but the experience may seem so unknown or daunting that they become frustrated and get stuck in the difficulty. To guide children forward in such situations means being with them in the moment of frustration and not shying away from it. Giving them the utter and complete assurance that you know they can do it. At times, it is not so easy to hold your ground with the child, as the difficulty and their frustration in that moment are very real, both emotionally and physically. It is a very special moment to be with a child when they are inside their frustration on the cusp of a breakthrough. It is a time of actively waiting for the child to move past their challenge and find their way to experiencing their new ability.

Moments of failure: These are frequently experienced by special needs children in therapeutic learning situations. Some children do not know they are failing, and others are all too aware of it. When learning something new, especially when there are objective challenges to be faced, there is, of course, no success without a certain amount of failure. Moments of failure shared with another person can either highlight and exaggerate the failure and render the experience a negative closing down time, or they may represent a moment of opening up into an experience of growth and new learning. A special needs child becomes a 'learner' when they experience each new moment of failure with an attitude of 'I want to try this again' or 'I can figure this out and do it.' Moments of failure are pivotal points in the development of a child, where confidence can either be instilled, or insecurity and fear can rise up and settle. How these moments are met by the child and the person guiding them helps to determine whether they will become magical miracle moments of ability or moments perceived as further proof of ineptitude.

Neuroplasticity, modifiability, and patterns of activity

We develop our identities to a large extent on the basis of interactions with our environment and the people in it. Identity development and interaction can only succeed if we feel perceived and accepted for the person we are. For children with special needs, it is especially important that their personality, potential, and abilities be kept in mind.

For therapeutic learning situations, this means

- reacting to the child with a certain spontaneity and orienting oneself toward the child;
- adapting the structure of the session to the neutral observations of the child's movements and behavior; and
- establishing contact with the child via playful interaction, suggesting adaptations, and promoting activity.

Due to their activating motoric and dynamic components, movement interactions can be particularly relevant for development and stimulate processes of learning, growth, and change.

6.1 Seeing the child as the person they are

When considering the timelines of a child's development, different methodologies and therapeutic learning systems have different ways of thinking about, approaching, and working with a child with developmental movement challenges. These different ways of thinking have important implications for the type of relationship one enters into with the child and how this relationship is used in a therapeutic learning process (Piek, 2006; Feldenkrais, 1977).

DOI: 10.4324/9781003737988-6

Deficit orientation: One of the ways of thinking about and relating to a child is via the diagnosis they have received. This includes a way of thinking that says there is something 'wrong' with the child and that this thing needs to be 'fixed.' Another way to say it would be that the child is faulty and needs to be repaired. Once fixed and repaired, the child will be normal and okay, but until then, there is something wrong. This creates a filter through which the child and any progress they make is viewed. It also presumes a direction of working with the child as though the child were an object. When a child is objectified, any manner of working with or relating to the child becomes acceptable—whatever is done and however it is done is justified, because the child needs it in order to be fixed, repaired, and made 'normal.' This may seem very unusual to some, but it is sadly very common. When speaking with parents, acquaintances, and professionals in the field, it may appear that they hold a different view, but upon delving more deeply, this deeply ingrained way of thinking often surfaces.

This framework of thinking and working relies on *comparisons* between atypically and typically developing children. It strives to turn the atypically developing child into something that they are not. The child is not seen for who and how they are, but rather as someone they should not be, because something is at fault with them. This places the child in a position where they are constantly judged against the background of who, what, and how they 'should' be and will be once the faulty aspects are mended. This also raises many expectations of the child, which, when unmet, reaffirm the thinking that something is 'wrong.' Has the repair work not yet been completed, or has the correct technique not yet been applied? When the child's movements are not performed 'correctly' or in the way they 'should' and 'need' to be, then the child must be 'corrected.' These corrections will be offered to the child over and over again, until they are done 'properly.' Only at that time will the child be worthy and okay. Consequently, only when the child becomes like a 'normal' child and moves in the 'correct' way—and only then—will such a way of thinking permit you to relate to them 'normally' and see them as the normal child they should and need to be. It places the burden on the child.

CASE EXAMPLE EMMA—BEHAVE AND MOVE UNEXPECTEDLY

The first impression upon meeting Emma was of a shy, withdrawn young girl. She would look up hesitantly for a brief moment and then back down at her toy, while holding on tightly to her parents and leaning into her father's leg. Emma seemed to be a bright, verbal child, yet whenever she spoke to her parents she would use a low voice, a kind of whisper.

When beginning to interact with Emma, everything needed to be completely calm and peaceful, or she would withdraw into herself even more. The voice had to keep a steady pace in a low, very relaxed tone. When any part of the situation and interaction moved too quickly for Emma, or she felt she was being pushed in any way to do something, play with something, or move in a particular way, she would immediately sink quickly back to sitting, lean on her parents, and lower her gaze.

Often, it takes time to get to know a child and the way they respond to the different types of interactions with all those present. Emma's parents would talk to her constantly and encourage her to cooperate. Yet it seemed as if they were not talking to Emma herself, but rather to her as though she were an object. It was as though they were talking to an imagined little girl that they wanted Emma to be, who needed to be directed to do any and every little movement or activity. They spoke as if they knew exactly how she should do everything in order to be 'healed,' 'corrected,' and 'fixed.' Emma was capable of moving in many ways, from being on the floor and sitting, up to standing and a type of walking with assistance. She had challenges with balance, her feet, the use of her hands, and a large degree of asymmetry between the sides of her body, resulting from damage to the brain that affects one side of the body more than the other. However, these didn't seem to be the main aspects hindering her progress. Emma was highly hesitant to move spontaneously or freely, or to do anything in the playful childlike manner one would expect in a 4-year-old. This appeared to have its roots in her worrying about doing everything incorrectly, wrongly, or not in the way her parents wanted.

It is important not to jump to conclusions about family dynamics. However, after repeatedly observing the behavior of the parents and Emma's way of responding to them in a number of sessions, it came across strongly that they did not see and/or relate to Emma as the sweet, intelligent child she is, who must deal with the objective developmental challenges she faces, but rather saw an object that just needed to learn how to do the right things in the right way.

In situations like this it can be a challenge to find the best strategy to 'get to' the child, particularly when anything Emma did was watched and monitored by her parents with a judgmental eye. During the first sessions, Emma began to notice that my way of being and doing things with her was different. There were no corrections to her actions, and when her parents pointed out a 'mistake,' I made light of it, as if to communicate to her that 'everything is okay,' 'it's no big deal,' 'you are fine.' This all needed to be done very carefully, so as not to give the parents the impression they were being contradicted in their parenting and relationship to Emma.

Slowly but surely, there emerged an encouraging type of playful silliness in our interactions and movements. The silliness was not one of being a clown, but rather an introduction to genuine childlike playful silliness, which promotes giggles and laughter and easy-going behavior, where there are no consequences if something does not go the way it was supposed to. In this way, an interactive wedge between Emma and her parents could be fostered. This allowed Emma to look out into the world toward me and see someone looking back at her in a way that allowed her to be as she was.

The transformation for her came at a moment which was shared between us, when she began to laugh uncontrollably, fell onto the floor, and started to roll around, kick, grab toys, and play. The out-of-control laughter lasted for well over five minutes. The expression on the parents' faces was one of bewilderment that their well-behaved little girl was out of control. At first, they told her to stop, but the situation was so genuine, and Emma was so engrossed in the feeling of herself and her own body, that the parents could not stop it and, eventually, became caught up in it. All joined in the laughter and playfulness of the moment.

From this point on, Emma transformed into a different girl. She was more daring and open to being guided into the world of play and learning. Progress was then possible in all the domains of balance and walking and use of her hands. She was able to focus on herself without the cautious, controlled behavior she had, in a sense, been indoctrinated into. It was evident that her parents loved her, yet they were functioning out of a mindset and strategy of fear, worry, and concern for their child. The discussions became very fruitful, and their entire relationship to Emma's challenges changed. It is often not the things we do, but the basis of our thinking that maintains the status quo and does not allow for progress.

Abilities orientation: Seeing the child for who they are creates a bridge; it enables us to relate to the child and their unique potentials and challenges. It requires a completely different paradigm and often an internal shift in thinking and perception. This paradigm looks at where the child is now on the developmental timeline. Abilities that are present and potentials not yet tapped are searched out. It sees the child as any other child, as a growing, developing person, with potential and many possibilities that can emerge if given the chance. The child is looked at from the perspective that a child deserves and needs encouragement, respect, and self-worth. The difficulties the child faces are viewed as challenges rather than problems. The practical applications of this paradigm shift are that you do what is needed at the time for the particular child to make progress, and not that which protocol dictates. The child is seen as completely normal for who they are, and not as a defective system needing to be fixed.

6.2 Foundations of a developmentally relevant therapeutic learning situation

Spontaneity, structure, and *interaction* are the foundations of a successful developmental therapeutic learning situation.

Spontaneity—orienting yourself toward others: All babies and young children have a natural, seamless behavioral flow during contact in relationships. They follow many nonverbal cues of whomever they are connecting and interacting with, and do not follow the conventional norms of social behavior that adults rely on. Babies and very young children do not yet have cultural norms of correct versus incorrect or good versus bad ways to interact or behave. This is also true, sometimes even more so, for an atypically developing child. The difference with many special needs children is that they tend to be somewhat more sensitive to new meetings and novel situations. But they are still children and will react in flow with you when you meet them if you behave in a non-threatening, open, authentic, and receptive way. For this to happen in a smooth manner, the session must begin spontaneously. It is important not to have a set plan when meeting the child and when the session starts. It is essential to begin by listening to the cues coming from the child, to react, and to observe how the child responds.

Structure—neutral observation: Initially, you must find a direction in which to interact such that the child does not feel threatened in any way. They can then begin to trust the new situation. Only now can touch and movement be initiated. If done too fast or rushed, there is the risk of losing the child's trust, and the effort made to establish a relationship will be fruitless. At the same time as establishing a trusting relationship, it is also important to make observations regarding how the child is moving, and whether they show interest in toys and in the surrounding social and physical environment.

By watching these movements and behavior, the initial structure of the session is established. It directs and gives an indication of what kinds of positions, movement relationships, and transitions are needed for the child to begin a process of learning change and further development.

Interaction—establishing contact playfully: Interactions are reciprocal in their nature. Knowing how to use the responses of the child to create communication on all levels, through and with the child's responses, facilitates the dynamics of the interaction (Siegel, 2007; Feldenkrais, 1981; Krauss, 1988; Knapp, Hall, & Horgan, 2007; Schore, 2019). How we respond while interacting can lead to new ways of acting and learning. Ways to begin to interact with the child while introducing movement elements are needed to keep and maintain the trusting relationship. Sequences initially performed in an exploratory and suggestive style lend the situation ease and a sense of not pushing oneself or the child in any specific direction. At the same time, the specific goals to strive toward should be kept in the foreground.

Learning and development are generally nonlinear. Learning, and particularly developmental learning, has rules of its own. These rules depend on a variety of considerations, including the specific age of the child and the type of developmental abilities and challenges that need to be addressed.

At any age or in any stage of a child's development, there must always be elements of play, surprise, challenge, success, and failure, as well as a large spectrum of emotions and sensations.

Interaction—suggest adaptations: Creating positive dynamic interactions through movement with a child assists them in developing more diverse and effective responses in movement as well as in their emotions, cognition, and sensations. It supports the child's regulatory process, which is itself an adaptive process responding to changing circumstances in the social and physical environment. With a special needs child, interactions may initially glean very little or no response at all. When the child's responses begin to appear, become more present, and, with time, fully recognizable, it is then possible to be more demanding and challenging in the interaction. How the child manages each new challenge is something to monitor very closely. As they begin to more easily manage a challenge that was once difficult or to which there was very little or an ineffective response, then it is possible to introduce challenges that are more complex and require more skill.

Interaction—promote activity: The majority of special needs children are left mostly alone with their developmental challenges during much of the day. In therapeutic situations, they are often put through regimes and set protocols which can be stressful and strenuous. Having a special needs child learn how to actively participate in a dynamic movement interaction is of great value for the child. The parts of the brain the child needs to be an active participant in their own developmental learning are aroused through these distinct, dynamic/animated interactions. In this way, opportunities are provided for active exploration, expression, and purposeful and functionally motivated action. The reactions and responses stimulate many vital parts of the nervous system involved in learning, which are not as frequently activated in special needs children because of the difficulties they face with being proactive in their own development.

6.3   Developmental movement interactions

Using interactions: There are many components of a developmental movement interaction. When implemented, they create an animated and stimulating setting for a child in which to learn, grow, and develop. They are spontaneous in character while at the same time very intentional and structured, with clear ideas and goals to move toward. The intention in the use of these components is to have these kinds of self and interpersonal behaviors emerge as developing skills and new abilities in the child. These skills and abilities will not become active without dynamic use. Activating them via interaction using the central tool of movement engages the brain in such a way as to simultaneously develop pathways to enrich other behavioral qualities. These pathways grow together based on the primary elements of movement, emotion, sensation, and the environment.

Examples of the animated qualities used in developmental movement interactions are

- meeting,
- following,
- leading,
- flowing with,
- suggesting/proposing,
- matching,
- pausing,
- listening,
- rhythms,
- speed,
- passive; active/pacing,
- resonating, dissonance, reconnecting,

- harmonizing,
- sharing moments,
- meshing,
- inquiring,
- questioning,
- challenging,
- demanding,
- integrating,
- giving attention to, and
- encouraging.

Meeting: The *meeting* is always the initial contact for each session and sets the tone for the dynamics of the interaction.

The children come in differently each day for each session. It is important to take the time to be clear and very attentive to the child, as this can make the difference between a productive and a nonproductive session. Meeting is the first interactive moment. To enter my private practice, you must first walk through a small garden and down a few steps. There are very large windows at the front of the practice through which I can see the family arriving and starting to descend the steps. If possible, I try to observe how the family approaches the steps and how they come down them. Who goes first? Are they talking together? Is the child being carried, are they smiling or clutching the parents? Are brothers or sisters or grandparents present, too? As I open the door to greet them, I observe and decide how best to meet and make initial contact with the child, the parent(s), and whomever else may be with them. Should I greet the child first or rather not look at the child and just talk to the parents? Often, I decide that it is best to make contact with the child first and then with the parents. However, I always base my decision on what I perceive to be best for the child in the specific moment, and not the cultural norm of who should be greeted first.

The type of initial contact is very important for the direction of the future relationship with the child. Should the meeting involve visual or verbal contact with the child, or perhaps neither? Waiting to see the expressions on the faces of all those coming down the steps, particularly the expressions and movements of the child, is a guiding factor. Is the child happy to be here and meet someone new? Or are they reluctant, curious, shy, fearful, sleeping, inattentive, or in any other state? A child is often timid or shy at the moment of meeting; they may have a toy they want to show, or they may not want to be here at all. However and whatever is present, being very alert to this and malleable enough not to miss either the subtle or the very obvious cues of the child—which can change at any moment—is essential. The children usually know they are coming to see me. I am always happy to see them and excited to meet a new child. The manner of 'acting' is by waiting to see the 'state' of the child and their initial responses to the new surroundings in that moment. Internal excitement does not always find outward expression. I always adjust my behavior to meet the child in the place they are in the moment they come. This 'meeting point' often sets a dynamic tone for the session.

Leading and following: As the session in movement begins, there is *following* and there is also *leading*. Following and leading are very different ways to interact with a child in movement. Following is when you don't want to interfere with the child but do want to let them know and sense, 'Ah! That person is going with me, they sense me, they feel me, they don't interfere.' Leading is when you say to the child, in a sense with your hands, 'I know you don't know what to do, but I'll take you there, we'll go together, I'll show it to you.' Flowing with is when there is no leader and no follower in the interaction, but there is a sense of fluidity. It feels effortless, a continuous back-and-forth interchange of leading and following.

Suggesting/proposing: It's not leading, it's not following; it's sort of like saying, 'Okay, would you like to try this? What do you think about that? Does this work?' You hint at something; this could be possible; maybe I'll follow if you start to go there; maybe you'll follow, and I'll lead you there.

Matching: In an interactive movement relationship, we have *matching*. This means you have to completely match the other person, become a match with them. Matching has many components: it means, 'We're here now together, me and you' and 'whatever we do, we do it together.' This requires special attention, because you have to approach the child, the child has to approach you, and there's a certain match—sometimes you have it, sometimes you don't.

Pausing: There are always elements of *taking pauses* in a session. Either you take a long pause and stop completely, or you're doing something and feel the child's not ready, you're too slow, or it's not right, so you just stop for a short moment, you pause, you wait, and then you continue.

Listening: Then there's an element of *listening*; listening to how the child moves, to how they feel when they move, listening for when there is a change, to the noises they make, listening to them, listening to the tone, listening to when the changes happen and how and where they happen, listening to whatever's present—and you have to listen with all your senses. Sometimes you're listening together, sometimes separately; the child may be listening to one thing, and you're listening to something else.

Rhythms: Each child has a different *rhythm*; each variety of muscular tone has a different rhythm of movement that accompanies them and which you can feel. Different kinds of movements have different rhythms. Rolling from the back onto the stomach or from the stomach onto the back are very different in terms of rhythm. Sitting up from lying on your back has a very different rhythm to lying down from sitting, and the rhythm of sitting to standing differs from that of standing to sitting.

Try it yourself—vary the speed, find the rhythm

Take any one or all of these examples and try them. Notice whether the rhythms are different and what you would have to do if you wanted to make them similar.

Notice how you roll from your back to your stomach and from your stomach to your back.

- Was it the same movement in reverse, or two different movements?
- Can you find a different way of rolling from your back to your stomach and from your stomach to your back?
- Can you change the rhythm of your movement at any point along the way?
- Is it easier to roll one way or the other, or in one of the variations you have chosen?
- Do you have a preferred way in which it is easier for you to control and vary the rhythm?

Once you have done this for rolling, try it for the other movements.

With a child you can let them set the rhythm, and you meet them, or you set the rhythm and see if the child meets it. Sometimes, finding the rhythm of how to make the movements happen allows the child to move. Sometimes it's making up a rhythm. Rhythms can vary depending on the movement, i.e., rhythms of rolling, rhythms in crawling, transitional rhythms, and static rhythms.

Speed: We all move at various *speeds* during our different daily activities, when we wake up, eat, or brush our teeth, or rush out of the house, exercise, etc.

For a child's growth, development, and experience of normal daily movement and activity, it is important that the child senses and feels and moves at different speeds. This will, of course, depend on the situation and condition of the child. Different developmental phases and stages need different speeds and rhythms in which to move.

If a child only experiences one way and one speed of movement, it is very difficult for the child and their musculoskeletal system to adjust to other rates of motion. Many factors need to be considered. For some children with spasticity, the rate of motion is critical for the initial learning of something new, as it is to the reaction of the spasticity in different movements.

Passive; active/pacing: Movements done *passively* are very different to movements done *actively* by the child, including the way in which they interact with the speed of the movement.

Resonating, dissonance, reconnecting, harmonizing: *Dissonance* can arise in many interactions. It arises when there is no matching, no shared rhythm; it doesn't work, it just doesn't come together. Something was wonderful, and then, all of a sudden, there's dissonance. Something happened; it's not working. Once there's dissonance, *how do you re-establish harmony?* Do you need to change the direction of the movement? Do you have to slow it down? Should you sing a song? Do you need to stop for a moment and remove your hands? Do you have to get up and let the mother take over the child? What can you do to recreate the harmony? Sometimes you're in one rhythm and the child's in another—how do you *harmonize the rhythms*, how do you play together in harmony?

Harmonizing and sharing moments: There are also sessions when there is complete *harmony*, and you *share moments* of movement, moments of emotion, of communication, of language; seeing things together, understanding a problem or an issue together. Sharing a moment with another human being in a harmonious way is a very powerful experience for child and practitioner. The child may not know it in the same way that you do, but they recognize that it's now with this other person, that the moment is shared.

Meshing: There's another aspect called *meshing*. Meshing differs from matching. Meshing is like when two fabrics intertwine, interlace, or become one unit; it just has a certain flow. This is special because there's a certain spontaneity that lets you feel you can just go and do things, because you are a single unit in the moment. You need to match before you can mesh.

Inquiring: *Inquiring* can be part of an interactive session. When you inquire, you try to find and figure out something about the child's movement. This can be done initially, when you begin to interact, or as part of the interaction. It can be done nonverbally and/or verbally. To inquire, one needs to be curious. Curiosity is a quality in an interaction that helps to remain neutral and non-judgmental. Inquiring is not done to find out whether something is good or bad; it is questioning and probing to see how something is moving and what the quality of a particular movement is. How are certain relationships of the movement fitting together, or how are they not? Is a movement clear for the child, or does some movement relationship require clarification? *Questioning* is more specific: how does this movement go, what does this muscle do, how is this joint, and what are the directions of the movement?

Demanding: Challenges and *demands* are essential. All children need challenges. Actually, everybody needs challenges. Without a certain amount of challenge, learning does not progress. It means that you want the child to accomplish something that you know can be done and is within the realistic reach of the child. It encroaches upon their comfort zone, but is not too far outside of it. You want the child to sense that they can do it. You want a positive challenge for the child, something that boosts their confidence. All children are different, and you can't challenge them too much; you can only challenge them with an amount they can manage and cope with on all levels. If it's too much, they don't know what to do and feel that they are being managed, pushed around, and asked to do something that has no connection to who they are. This is to be avoided, as it is something that can be prominent in the foreground of a special needs child.

Demanding is very different to challenging. Demanding is: 'You're going to do it, and I know you can.' You cannot demand of all children. Yet it is legitimate and can be a very useful and effective part of a session. To demand from a child, you must know that they can do what you are asking of them, that they are physically and emotionally ready and able to do it in that particular moment. You must also be very clear with yourself and know how to specifically guide the child toward fulfilling your demand. Demanding is not an easy thing to do, but at the right moment and with the right force, it can bring extraordinary results. Being able to *clarify* how something moves, i.e., the direction of the movement, the quality, an angle, a position, a transition, or a relationship, is a vital part of the dynamics of an interaction.

Integrating: Then there's the component of *integrating*. Integrating comprises bringing together many elements of a relationship or pattern of movement and behavior after clarifying each part separately. An example of this could be when learning how to roll onto the back from sitting by way of the side. There are many single elements of this pattern. A few are tilting the head back and forth so that the balance shifts to one side, lifting and side-bending of one side of the pelvis for shifting the weight, leaning onto the palm of the hand to accept the weight, bending of the elbow to lean over, and going down onto the forearm. All these elements contribute to a full pattern of a transitional movement from sitting to lying on the back. It is accomplished in a leaning and rolling onto the side movement, and then from the side onto the back. Each element has parts that need to be learned individually. Integrating is when all of the singular parts of the movement are put together to form one entire pattern of movement.

Try it yourself—integrating movement patterns

Take a moment to try this out.

- Sit comfortably on the floor with your knees bent to the sides and the soles of your feet facing one another. From this starting position, go through each of the elements described above separately. Try not to do it as an 'exercise' but rather with the attitude that you are setting out to notice something new about this kind of movement and learn something from it.
- Once you have done each part separately, begin to combine them. Go back and forth between the individual parts until the full pattern of movement becomes clear and smooth.
- Once you have done this, think for a moment what it would be like to interact with someone else in movement, and nonverbally and interactively guide them through the individual elements and, ultimately, toward integration of them all into the entire pattern.
- Now imagine doing the same thing with a special needs child. A child who has never done this movement may possibly be nonverbal, and who has challenges in some aspects, be they in balance or control over their limbs, or spasticity or low tonus.

Encouraging: Interacting by *encouraging* a child during a developmental learning session is a component that can be very useful. Any child, typically or atypically developing, needs encouragement and has a special feeling when they are encouraged. Many special needs children are not certain of the importance or the meaning of what they are doing or of why it is important for them do certain things that they don't do on their own.

When there is a specific part of a movement the child is having difficulty with, or in a situation in which they may be struggling to repeat something or move in a particular direction that is unknown or creates uncertainty, a very specific moment of encouragement can make a world of difference. Interactive encouragement does not have to be through words only. It can be offered by singing, through a different tone of a sound, by using emphasis in the hands leading the child, or while following them. It can, of course, also be conveyed in words. Different cultures have different ideas regarding the use of encouragement in therapeutic learning situations. I have always found it very useful to encourage the child, no matter what culture they are from. When offered at the right moment, in the right intensity, and in a dynamic interactive manner, encouragement can have profound and positive effects on the child.

6.4   Promoting neuroplasticity through learning and activity

Not so long ago, the idea of neuroplasticity was not widely acknowledged. Nowadays, the concept of plasticity in the brain and nervous system is well recognized and has been intensively studied and researched. With the introduction of plasticity, new, wide-ranging directions have opened up in the understanding of learning, growth, development, and change. These ideas are also increasingly accepted in experiential and therapeutic learning situations.

Neuroplasticity: Plasticity means that the nervous system has the capacity to change and reorganize throughout life, by forming and strengthening neural connections both functionally and structurally (Konner, 2010; Siegel, 1999). These changes come about in response to and as a result of personal experience. Neural plasticity also allows the brain to counteract and possibly offset the effects of various altered directions of growth and development in functional movement. These alterations may be due to, e.g., injury, deficiency, or genetic variations. Neural plasticity unlocks the potential for neurons and neural networks to adjust and adapt their activities in response to newly encountered experiences and situations, as well as to changes in their environment.

Modifiability: The ideas, concepts, and applications of neural modifiability are relevant to both typically and atypically developing children, as well as to adults. There are numerous ways to bring plasticity into action through movement.

Another way to express plasticity in relation to the nervous system and brain is the ability of the nervous system to modify itself and change, including the way in which it achieves this. This neuromodifiability depends on the ways in which the brain and the nervous system interact with the environment and the people within it. Applying the ideas of plasticity to learning through personal experience is both stimulating and challenging.

Use it or lose it: The most basic of all applications is represented by the well-known expression 'use it or lose it.' Practically, this means that if you don't continue to use an ability or practice it in certain activities, the ability has no means of growing and developing and may be lost altogether. This also implies that not only the specific ability at hand can be lost, but also that all the interconnections that this ability had, would, or could have formed can be lost too. *Skills* that are infrequently applied are most likely to vanish over time. For a special needs child, this has great implications. A special needs child often does not or cannot use an ability or certain movements and configurations without external facilitation. It is thus very important that the child be assisted to use specific movements, so that these can begin to appear in their movement repertoire and become represented in their brain. This also applies to movements which are present in the child's repertoire but difficult for the child to perform on their own, so that they do not disappear.

Practice and 'using' what is done with the child can be of great help in furthering progress, to ensure that it is not lost between sessions. 'Use it or lose it' need not only apply to the movements themselves, but also to the way in which they are performed, as well as to the approach to their use:

- use it in a way that brings pleasure and not pain,
- use it so it becomes a process to follow,
- use it so that it allows for exploration,
- use it in a way that does not force the child but rather encourages them and arouses their curiosity, and
- use it in a way that provides new varieties of speeds and pauses.

Use it and improve it: Another idea of neuromodifiability is 'use it and improve it.' This encompasses learning that drives and pushes forward a specific function to help enhance it. This means that if a child has some ability in a phase of movement, i.e., some form of crawling already developed, albeit not particularly smooth or coordinated, or if the child is able to be upright and take steps, but they continue to be hesitant, using the particular function specifically can improve it. Crawling can be used to learn more about crawling and to improve crawling. Sitting can be improved by sitting. Walking can be improved in walking, etc.

This also implies that once the pleasurable / explorative / non-forced / curiosity-awakening manners of use are implemented, that these internal aspects of actional experiences can be improved upon. This improves not just the action itself, but also the process of learning the action.

Repetition: In facilitating neuromodifiability, repetition is vital to create the possibility for change to take hold. Beginning a process of modification and change for a specific ability, e.g., rolling onto the stomach, lifting the head to the horizon while on the stomach, or coming onto the hands and knees, requires ample repetition. The specific manner of repetition is also relevant to the learning and neuromodification process. The outcome will show whether the most effective and useful strategy has been used for the child; if one approach is ineffective, another should be tried.

Specificity and variability: Some children need to have specific movements repeated in exactly the same order and sequence in which they were presented each and every time, otherwise the learning does not take hold. Other children frequently need to have the order and sequence changed and not repeated in the same way. There are also children who need a varied combination of both tactics. Whereas there are short-term changes that can be seen in children, our real interest is in these changes taking hold and becoming long-term changes. Repetition is a necessary part of helping short-term changes turn into long-term changes. It fosters progression in the learning of new skills and abilities, from the initial phase of learning to an automatic action pattern.

The importance of timing and age: The younger one begins, the better; the more age- / ability-appropriate the action, the better. Neural modifiability is more probable and possible the earlier it is started with special needs children. Younger brains are more amenable to the process of change. Introducing different strategies of plasticity that facilitate the growth and development of movement learning early on will have a better chance of forming strong connections. The earlier the better, so that unformed patterns of movement and activity can be introduced, practiced, and learned. Neural networking that assists in the child's voluntary movement and behavior can be more easily formed at an age- or ability-appropriate time, depending on the developmental timeline of the individual child.

Intensity of the challenges and tasks: All children need and thrive on the basis of challenges in the learning process. While the challenge should not be beyond their level of competence in movement, cognition, or emotion, it must arouse and motivate them enough to work toward arriving at something new. They need to sense and feel that they can do it, that they can accomplish something new if they take hold and try. A demand made of a child must be presented in such a way that the child feels that they can do it. This requires a certain degree of insistence, but not so that the child is overwhelmed or loses self-confidence or self-trust. The opposite needs to be gauged for the challenge: if the 'size' of the challenge is gauged well, then the child will gain self-confidence, self-trust, and feel that they can manage and deal with greater challenges more easily. This elicits a modification in the child's ability to accept new and more demanding situations of movement, emotion, sensation, and learning.

Relevance: The information and movement must be relevant to the child. If not, a way to find relevance must be sought. Some sort of emotional connection for the child involved in the movement, action, or activity will have a greater chance of conveying relevance, so that the process of neural modifiability proceeds more fluidly and effectively. The child's skill level, disposition, and temperament toward certain movements must also find relevance in and connection to the child's environment.

Transference and integration of learned abilities: Elements of developmental movement sequences and patterns can be used partially or fully in other sequences or patterns in other positions in gravity. Elements of coming to sit can be used in learning how to come onto one knee and foot or to stand. Patterns within sitting can be implemented in learning how to roll from the stomach to the back. The information and type of movement can be interchanged, transferred, and integrated into other developmental sequences. The particular movement, e.g., coming to sit, might not be fully formed, but movements and patterns further along on the developmental pathway may be. Elements from these more developed patterns can be used to assist further development and learning of earlier ones.[1]

Note

1   The ideas of use it or lose it, use it and improve it, specificity, repetition matters, intensity matters, time matters, age matters, and transference are based on Kleim, J. A., & Jones, T. A. (2008). Principles of Experience-Dependent Neural Plasticity: Implications for Rehabilitation after Brain Damage. *J Speech Lang Hear Res.*, *51*(1): 225–239. doi:10.1044/ 1092-4388(2008/018).

Freedom in movement 7

Movement organization is highly individual. The therapeutic goal is to accompany the child toward playful discovery and development of their own organization, efficiency, and clarity in movements that are purposeful and controlled. Exploratory learning and sensory perceptions can be important means to establish contact to oneself and to others. An expanded freedom of movement paves the way toward new possibilities of verbal and non-verbal communication and development of emotional skills.

7.1 Play, chaos, and movement organization

Efficient movement organization: There is chaotic organization of movement and there is efficient organization of movement. When movement is efficiently organized it feels easy, smooth, and flowing; real-izing one's intentions—what one wants to do, where one wants to go, and how to get there—is uncomplicated. Chaotically organized movement is uneven, rough, problematic, effortful, and demanding. It does not carry through to the intended goal or misses it, is problematic and lacks struc-ture (Feldenkrais, 1981; Van der Kolk, 2012; Edelman, 2001; Schonkoff & Phillips, 2000).

An efficiently organized pattern of movement does not usually draw our attention unless we are watching a sporting or dance event. The more effi-ciently organized the movement, the more our attention is drawn to the particular player or dancer. We notice the ones who exhibit extraordinary organization in sport, dance, and theater. They stand out and we are drawn

DOI: 10.4324/9781003737988-7

to them and in awe of them. We emulate them and how they perform their art or sport. When a movement has a chaotic organization, it stands out, too. We tend to notice it more. The more chaotic, the more it draws our attention.

During the process of typical development, we see the spontaneous, structured, and efficient organization of movement emerge during the child's first years. More and more abilities form and appear. The child has more and more intentions and discovers more efficient ways to realize and accomplish their needs and interests.

Chaotic movement organization: Chaotic organization of movement is very often seen in special needs children and can be observed in different ways. It can be seen in the effort needed to move in certain directions, or while a child is trying to accomplish a certain movement, and something else takes place every time. Take a child with a spastic arm and hand, for example. They may have the intention to reach out and grab an object and can assess where it is, but because of the spasticity, each time they try to reach out, the hand and arm become spastic, and the arm goes somewhere else. The movements may be uncontrollable, as in children with dystonia. The movement may be chaotic because it is too demanding due to a lack of strength. The skeleton may collapse or go in directions that don't transmit the forces in a way that maintains a clear or straight direction. Or a reflex takes over when the child wants to roll, and instead of rolling, the head goes one way and the shoulder and arm the other.

CASE EXAMPLE ALEX—CLARIFYING INDIVIDUAL MOVEMENT ORGANIZATION

Alex was a very expressive child but could not speak and say what he wanted. When he attempted to do any movement in any direction on his own, the movements were done with great force, exhibiting chaos in terms of direction and intention. When observing Alex move, it was very difficult to understand what he was trying to accomplish, what movement he was trying to do, or where he wanted to move.

All of Alex's movements were very fast and done with tremendous muscular strength. Although nonverbal, he was very interactive and communicative. He wanted to express himself and be a part of his surroundings. He would initiate contact, make lots of sounds in different tones, and contort his face, trying to communicate with whatever means he had.

When most people heard and looked at Alex, it would seem that his movements had no sense or order, and that he was just making loud, nonsensical noises. However, when I looked at Alex, I saw a child struggling to move in the ways he wanted but being overcome by the neurological challenges of his system. His muscles were held very tight, and his joints were positioned in different directions. Alex was very friendly and interested in making contact. The objective when helping him was to give him a secure, calm feeling, and create a clear order of different movements, so that he could follow with his attention when someone else was 'doing the movements for him.' In this way, Alex would have the opportunity to listen unhindered by his own system, to let him understand where it was possible to move and make sense of it. If Alex could fully trust the person acting as his external guide, and provided the directions and order of the movements were absolutely clear, then he would have a means of making internal sense and order of the movement. This would assist him in clarifying his own intention and become more able to initiate and follow through with his movements. Maintaining a constant verbal connection with him was essential, even though our mother tongues were different.

I wanted to show and guide Alex, with my hands, through the specific set of movements that he needed and could follow to understand more clearly how to roll himself from his back, onto his side, and then onto his stomach, and return. At first, the strength in his muscles would not abate, but after more repetitions performed in an easy-going, light, and gentle manner, his entire system slowed down to allow all the specific movements in a very clear way, so that he could sense, feel, and move through the configurations. The order needed to be kept constant, repetitive, and clear.

The sessions with Alex took place in front of a group. As it turned out, he loved the attention and seemed to very much enjoy being the center of attention. When he was guided gently and clearly, his entire system would gradually slow down and begin to soften. A very special look would come into his eyes, a look of extraordinary calmness and fascination at what was being done.

After 30 minutes, it was time to stop and leave Alex to himself. He would lie quietly for a few moments, absorbed in the new sensations within himself. Then, from one second to the next, he would recommence his fast and forceful movements. When the participants looked at Alex, they were all enrapt to see that even though his movements were still forceful, jerky, and strong, it was possible to tell that he was re-enacting all the movements that he had been guided through while in a calm state. He did not follow the smooth order of the movements exactly, but it was evident that he was now searching for each of them and trying to have his intention and new understanding fit together within the objective challenges of his musculature and skeleton. He became more and more expressive and vocal, and managed to roll very clearly from his back, onto his side, onto his stomach, and back again. Each time one of his movements succeeded for him in a way that rolled him further, he beamed out happiness and satisfaction, expressing loudly to the group in his own unique way, 'Look at me! I can do it now!' 'I did it!' 'I can!'

His special way of doing things was present, and the neurological aspects that put extraordinary demands on his system were also present, but now, through all of this, he could make sense and create an intention of movement and bring it to realization.

New movement organization through play: To assist a special needs child in formulating a clearer and less chaotic understanding of itself in movement, a very particular mode of play is used to interact with the child.

At different ages, children engage cognitively as well as emotionally in different forms of play. Early on, they play with and by themselves, and slowly progress to active and interactive participation with others. This contact and interaction allows for a variety of types of interactive modes, and not just what can be thought of as a typical therapeutic approach focused directly on results and making great demands of the child. Play permits an environment for the child in which the means are prominently in the foreground, and the ends are in the background. Both means and ends are very important for a special needs child. Challenges in the use of their bodies can make it very difficult for a special needs child to initiate and sustain acts of play, either by themselves or together with someone else.

Engaging in play activity passively or actively is also a means and an end in itself. Play has a special function in the development of the brain. Through detailed interactive play with a special needs child, it is possible to put specific parts of the chaos in their movements into clear focus. Once this focus appears, it is then possible to engage in a process of framing the chaos. In this playful manner, the focus is directed toward the specifics of particular movements which are needed to assist the child in creating order and efficiency. The play is spontaneous, and the movements are presented in a structured, random manner around the particular functional movement ability that needs more order. By proceeding in this fashion, there is a certain degree of mimicking the process by which a typically developing brain achieves a complex, efficient organization of its movement and actions.

Let individual order appear: The above-described type of play enables the child to engage in a focused manner without needing or having knowledge of the success or failure of what they are or should be doing. It is a systemic way of approaching the chaos found in the movements of a special needs child. When you offer the particular elements that the child needs to fit together in a random yet structured way, this enables more efficient organization and allows a less chaotic order of movement to emerge more easily and quickly.

No one can create order or organization in the movements of a child. It is the child's brain itself that creates the change. The job of the therapeutic practitioner is to create an environment of play and offer the movements in a random yet structured manner, so that the brain has what it needs to create order out of the chaos.

7.2   Exploration and discovery as primary elements of therapeutic learning

Exploratory learning of sensory perception: Exploration and discovery of one's Self, one's body, and one's spatial environment is a primary activity in early development (Fogel, 2013; Feldenkrais, 1981). It is instrumental in development of the sensory, movement, cognitive, and emotional world of a child. Through movement, touch, and smell, the infant innocently explores its own body, others, and the surrounding environment. At first, this happens in a haphazard, indiscriminate fashion: finding the mouth and fingers; sensing the interconnection of fingers and hands; the discovery of one's own face, mouth, eyes, nose, ears, and hair. Moving hands and fingers away from the central part of the body and then moving them closer once again. Sensations of the feet and toes touching while sliding a foot along the other leg. Crossing an arm over the body from one side to the other and reaching out for something.

Being able to use the hands to bring something into the mouth seems so simple that we take it very much for granted. Think of how many of the activities that we perform daily involve the use of the hands in conjunction with other parts of the sensorimotor system.

During the first months of life, a baby begins to be able to make use of their hands, mouth, and eyes. They use these for exploring and understanding themself, other people, the environment, and objects. Soft, hard, rough, smooth, wet, dry, hot, cold, slimy, mushy, squishy, near, far, pleasant, unpleasant, light, heavy, solid, and liquid are just a few of the sensations and consistencies we encounter with fingers, hands, and other parts of the body. After a period of time, we learn to interpret what we have touched and gain the ability to recognize it visually and know what to expect when we encounter it again.

Objects need to be touched and explored numerous times before the consistency is clearly recognizable. Smell, touch, and the visual system are engaged in most of these explorations simultaneously. When grabbing, pushing, and pulling begin to become part of the exploration and discovery process, the sense of weight, distance, and force used is felt, calculated, and ascertained. Understanding the distance we need to cover to take something when it is not directly next to us is also part of this exploration and discovery process.

When turning the focus to a special needs child, the impact of exploratory learning of sensations of weight, distance, consistency, texture, etc. can be appreciated. It is enough to think of a young spastic or hypotonic child who has either too much tone in their hands and cannot bring them to their mouth or touch and explore any part of their body, or too little tone to lift and move their arms.

Understanding with the hands: It is essential to create processes of exploration and discovery and offer these to a child in therapeutic learning situations. Not only do they help in the movement and sensory domains, but they also help either passively or actively in the child's cognitive development. The hands are a primary source of understanding, knowledge, and expression. A child who never has the use of their hands and fingers as a tool of exploration, manipulation, and expression misses out on a large portion of developmental learning and growth.

CASE EXAMPLE DANIEL—DISCOVERING ONE'S OWN LIMBS WITH CURIOSITY

Daniel was a 6-year-old boy with spastic cerebral palsy. His hands were bent and twisted in such a way that only the back of the wrist and forearm were visible to him, and his fingers were closed in a fist-like position with the thumb on the inside. He was unable to open his hands or move his fingers because of the position they were constantly held in. Daniel was a nonverbal child with big, wide eyes and a cheerful demeanor. He was attentive and communicative.

Daniel's back was well enough developed, with sufficient strength and tone to maintain a sitting position with his feet on the floor. If he leaned too much to the left or right, he would begin to lose balance. His reactions were timely, and he would quickly and effectively put the back of his hand and wrist onto the table to regain himself and return to sitting upright. For him, this was his hand and how he had taught himself to use it. It was clear that he had the ability and understanding to control elements of his movements; however, for some reason, Daniel had never had the opportunity to learn how to use his hands and fingers in such a way that his fingers and wrists could turn and open. Thinking about what kind of representation and internal image in terms of sensation and movement he had developed for his hands and fingers over the course of six years was intriguing, as he had developed use of them while they were maintained in a constant twisted and closed position.

Beginning to turn the forearm in directions that also allowed movement in the shoulder joint was agreeable to him. From there, it was possible to turn, twist, bend, and begin to straighten his wrist. His expression when this was done was one of utter fascination. Slowly but surely, over the course of a few sessions, it was possible to show Daniel how to bring the palm of his hand up to contact the side of his face. The first time this exploratory movement was performed, it needed to be done passively. His reaction was as though someone else was touching him, and he did not know who it was or why it was being done. He seemed to be a bit anxious and taken aback by what was happening. Only when it became feasible to show him his hand in an exploratory way, so that he could look directly at it in front of him and actively take part in turning his own forearm, hand, and wrist—once to the back side of the hand and once to the palm—did he come to actually recognize it as his hand. This discovery and recognition of his own hand paved the way to allowing his hand to touch his cheek without hesitation or caution. For Daniel, this initially passive and later active curious exploration of his own cheek and face represented a new part of himself opening up and the doorway to an explosion of interest in the use of his hands and discovery of his fingers. His spasticity did not disappear, but by being able to be moved through the required directions of movement, at first passively, in an agreeable and pleasant way, he was able to develop sensation of the movements needed to control and use his hands, wrists, and fingers more actively and in many more ways than before.

7.3   The joy of new freedom in movement

Challenges and frustration: Many special needs children have challenges and difficulties in movement. They can become frustrated when trying to accomplish sequences such as reaching, rolling onto the side, crawling forward, or standing up from a chair and walking. They may have the interest and motivation to move, but their intentions are realized only partially or not at all (Figure 7.1). Perhaps they try something and even have the correct idea of what to do, but the connection between their brain and the endpoint in their musculoskeletal system receives a different message. Some special needs children cannot repeat the same movement twice in the same way. Each attempt—even with a clear idea and intention of what they want to accomplish—has a different result. This is highly frustrating for the child. This frustration can be compounded if they feel misunderstood, and may even turn to anger. How, as an adult with our sense of Self, could we possibly understand what it is like not to be able to accomplish a simple thing we take for granted, no matter how hard we try or how many attempts we make?

Joy and self-efficacy: The joy and elation that is felt when a new freedom of movement and ability is perceived is one of the greatest experiences a child with special needs can have. They become so happy, sometimes even giggling hysterically with joy. It is a wonderful experience to be part of, to witness the new vitality with new connections being established in the brain and body. The more frequently a child has these kinds of experiences, the more they build in the child a sense of 'I am,' 'I am capable,' 'I can do it,' 'I want to.' Thousands upon thousands of neural connections are buzzing with new life in the child's brain, connecting to one another and becoming stronger and stronger together.

The joy that is experienced in more freedom of motion helps to improve the child's relationship with their Self. It promotes an overall feeling in the child of becoming more and more themself in the world of movement, and furthers their sensation of being an autonomous person.

Some moments of elation stem from very small new connections, accomplishments, and curiosities, others from large breakthroughs. Yet the more these elements and the emergence of basic building blocks—small or large—are encouraged, the more the child finds themself on a continuum of progress, evolution, and improvement; the more the child feels and senses that they can, and not that they cannot.

Feeling joy in movement communicates to the child's entire image of their Self that the direction in life is one of ability, possibility, and freedom, and not of difficulties, problems, and inability. The child's self-perception

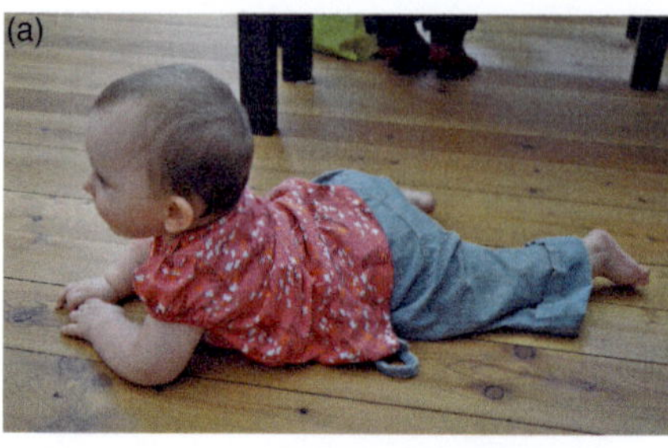
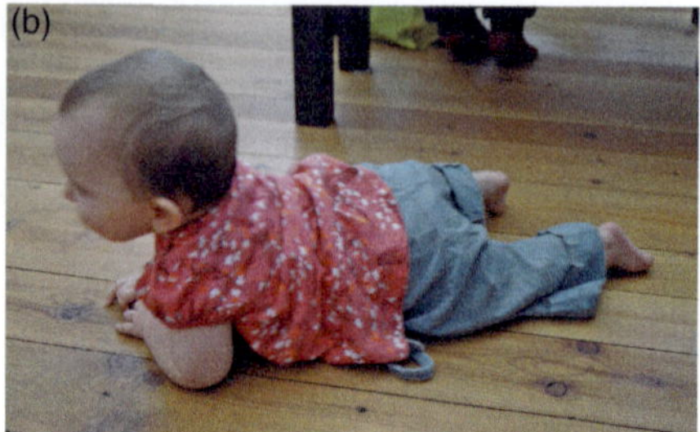
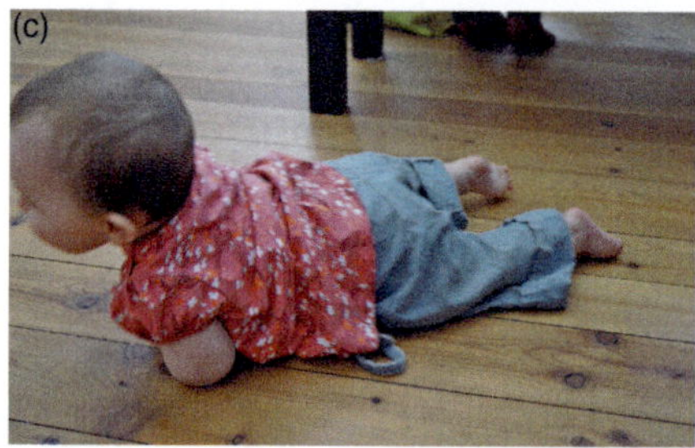

Figure 7.1: Forward motion on the elbows and forearms

can change from 'I cannot.' 'I will never be able to.' 'I am not worth it!' to 'I did it!' 'I can!' 'I am of value!'

Self-worth, self-value, self-esteem, and pride are not only psychological states, but they are also neurobiological imperatives. They are strong positive forces for encouraging interest in more freedom and joy in motion in the child. This is taken for granted when considering the developmental direction of a typically developing child, and the idea must be transferred to the domain of special needs children—both in theory and in practice.

What is of significance to observe in the three photos of the child shown in Figure 7.1 is the interplay between the positions of the left elbow and forearm, the left shoulder joint, and the head. The child is using the left forearm and elbow to pull and move themself forward.

In photo a), the left elbow and forearm are in front of the left shoulder joint, and the head is upright and behind the elbow and forearm.

In photo b), the positions of the forearm, elbow, head, and shoulder joint have changed. The forearm and elbow are directly under the shoulder joint, and the head is further forward and above the left shoulder joint, elbow, and forearm.

In photo c), the left elbow and forearm are behind the left shoulder joint, and the head is in front of the left shoulder joint, elbow, and forearm.

7.3.1 Nonverbal communication and self-regulation

Communicating nonverbally: Finding ways to regulate ourselves is something learned in early life through and with another person. As infants, we need someone to help us regulate almost everything: our heart rate, breathing rhythms, sleeping, and eating. We also need someone to regulate our moods and rhythms of activity. As infants, we need support and regulation in the ways we connect to others, including how we come into contact, maintain contact, and reconnect when the connection is lost (Schore, 1994; Feldenkrais, 1981; Hüther, 2006, 2018). As infants, we communicate our needs nonverbally, as we have no way to communicate verbally before the age of at least 18 months. During this early period of life, children express their needs nonverbally. An attuned parent or caregiver knows how to listen to these nonverbal cues and knows how to respond and meet the needs being communicated. The communication is through sound, facial expressions, and body language. Even once a child has learned to communicate verbally, they will continue to also communicate nonverbally in many ways throughout life; this is a continuous part of daily waking life.

Feeling nonverbally understood: Special needs children also communicate nonverbally (Knapp, Hall, & Horgan, 2007). Their bodies frequently do not do what they want them to do, which makes clear communication in the nonverbal domain more challenging. Being able to listen to a special needs child in the nonverbal domain, to hear the child and respond to their needs, is a gift to a special needs child. They feel listened to, known, seen, and included. Being listened to and heard by someone when they express themselves in their own unique way is a concrete sensory experience for the special needs child. This person knows them and is listening. As adults, we have all had the experience, with an intimate partner or close family member or friend, that when something is troubling us deeply, and our entire being is saying so nonverbally, we want, need, and assume that this person is able to 'listen' to what we are saying without us having to put it into words. There is the feeling that if it needs to be verbalized, it lowers the value, because 'they should know without us having to say it.' If they see us and know us, they 'should' understand what we are communicating without words.

Establishing contact through movement: This is why it is so important for us to know how to listen to the needs of our own bodies and to know how, as adults, to regulate many facets of our internal and external selves. One way to do this is to learn how to listen to our needs in movement, and to be with ourselves in the nonverbal domain of internal, beyond-words communication. We often have many internal conversations when we try to be quiet by ourselves. When entering the sensorimotor domain of self-listening and self-learning through movement, we acquire a very different and important way to pay attention to another part of ourselves. This improved sense of one's own needs in movement—of how to make oneself feel good through movement, of how to listen to one's needs—is a major component of how we 'connect' through movement to a special needs child.

Communicating through movement: When this connection is via the nonverbal medium of movement, it has a potent, profound, and important effect on both the system of the child as well as our own. Having the child feel pleasant sensations through movement wakes up parts of their brain that release chemicals which produce positive sensations. For the brain to develop in a productive manner, these sensations need to be at very high levels during the formative years. A special needs child needs another person to achieve this, as their body cannot and does not do it on its own, in the manner of a typically developing child. This is an ability of the brain and of the Self (Ellingsen et al., 2016).

Losing the connection to and reconnecting with ourselves and others in early life, as well as understanding our emotions and the meaning of our emotions, is accomplished through and with another. We all lose our self-balance and must learn ways to return to it. When we are off base in any way, we recognize it in ourselves and in our bodies. Once we have learned to connect with ourselves, we can find ways to return, to feel more connected to ourselves, and, in turn, to others. In early life, we learn to feel through and with another the sense of this connection and the sense of ourselves, of who and how we are. When we lose this, we seek out those who can help us to regain this sense of ourselves. This sense of Self is a body-based sensory emotional experience. It resides in all our senses, and we know how to recognize it. It is internalized very early on. When our own self-regulation is too far off, we may seek professional help (Heller & LaPierre, 2012; Hüther, 2006; Krauss, 1988; Schore, 2012; Feldenkrais, 1985).

7.3.2 Developing emotional abilities through interaction and movement

Emotions and feelings: Emotional learning also takes place during a therapeutic learning session. An integral part of an interactive learning situation is the way the child's movements and emotions interact with another person. Emotions are interpersonal and interrelational (Stern, 1985; Hüther, 2006;

Krauss, 1988; Van der Kolk, 2012). Emotions are physical manifestations. They are neurophysiological reactions in response to external and internal stimuli. Emotional life is associated with a large variety of continuous bodily reactions and adjustments. Self-perception and the personal experience of our emotions culminate in what we call feelings (Damasio, 2010)

Emotional learning: Very early on in infancy, emotional learning occurs via interactions with primary caregivers and other family members. Much of very early emotional learning is also culturally dependent. As the child grows, the circle of social–emotional interactions also grows. In interactive learning situations, these interconnected elements help the child to discover how to be attentive to themselves and what they are feeling. It is another direction of getting to know themselves with and through their emotions. This, in turn, assists them in finding ways to understand themselves and interpret the social interactions and engagements they are involved in during interactive learning through movement. When changes in the child's movement take place and movements become easier, more feasible, and pleasant, they also have a clear effect on the child's emotional regulation.

Mirroring learning experiences: Echoing a child's emotional state back to them in an interactive movement learning experience is an important but difficult task. It is achieved through a collaborative reaction and interaction that takes place simultaneously with the changes that are happening during the moments of the movements with which the interaction is engaged. This helps the child establish a new connection with themself. The child directly and animatedly experiences their own emotions, while at the same time sensing their unique way of performing a movement and being in contact with another person. This is a complex, multifunctional developmental task. For this type of learning interaction to be effective, a high level of attention is demanded of the child and a high level of skill of their interaction partner.

Interaction with variation: Introducing variations to the interaction in the movements, including varying the emotional tone and flow of the inter-action, allows for growth in the child's interactive behavior and in their devel-opment of social contact and interfacing. It gives the child a better sense of their Self. Many special needs children do not have as wide a repertoire of behavioral interactive skills as typically developing children. This may simply be due to the limited number of children with whom they meet and have the opportunity to relate to and interact with. Increased self-attention, mindfulness, and experience of their emotional Self and feelings can foster further growth and development in the child's communication skills. To be heard and understood in an interaction—nonverbally or verbally—is vital for any child and even more so for a child with special needs.

7.3.3   Dealing with unpleasant past experiences

Respect negative experiences: Any and all new situations that resemble a previous unpleasant experience will often evoke hesitancy, anxiety, and apprehension in a child. Some special needs children have suffered from unpleasant experiences from a very early age. This may have been initially in the hospital or with primary caregivers, or because they have undergone therapies that do not take into consideration the possible discomfort for the child. Some have been handled in very unpleasant and sometimes painful ways. This renders the child justifiably anxious, hesitant, apprehensive, on-guard, and suspicious of any new situation with an adult.

Provide positive experiences: It is essential to understand and appreciate how these previous experiential encounters shape the reactions and responses of a child. It is a gift to a child who has had previous unpleasant experiences— and to their family—when you give them a positive and pleasant experience in a therapeutic learning situation. This is of the highest priority and is at the core of my thinking, way of working, and teaching. It is important to keep this in mind when meeting a child, and you must find ways to implement it. The value of pleasant positive experiences cannot be underestimated, neither in the short nor in the long term. The whole nervous system responds in a completely different way when it has repeated pleasant experiences compared to when it has repeated unpleasant or painful ones (Feldenkrais, 1972; Stern, 1985; Heller & LaPierre, 2012; Hüther, 2006; Van der Kolk, 2012; De Waal, 2009). This topic is coming more and more into the foreground of therapeutic learning and care. The understanding and acceptance that positive experiences in all aspects of learning and care have a profound impact on outcomes related to learning, growth, and development of the child—physically, emotionally, and mentally—is, happily, increasing.

CASE EXAMPLE MATTHEW—BEING IN A SAFE PLACE

Matthew is a very communicative nonverbal child. Upon first meeting him, my impression was of a child with little tone and little or no control. He had many repetitive hand movements that he would often resort to. From what I had been told, Matthew had had many very difficult and unpleasant experiences before arriving in my office. My initial impressions were that movement-wise, it would not be a difficult task to work with Matthew. My concern was on the emotional side, of being able to make contact with Matthew and have him feel completely safe and secure at each and every moment. This required me to be extremely slow and acutely attentive to every minute aspect of everything I did with him. I had never had a child who required such extreme attention to every change of movement, to every type of touch and tone and rhythm of voice.

Matthew would often make sounds of various kinds. Sometimes as if to communicate and say something, and other times there seemed to be no sense to his sounds and their pitch. If something was in any way disagreeable to him, he would break out into a heartfelt crying spell and would need time with his parents to bring him back into a calm state. It could be the type of touch, whether firm or soft, steady or hesitant. It could be the direction being moved in or the position in space. Often, it was hard to decipher what would disturb him and have him retreat and become so agitated. Each time this happened, I would have to start as if from the very beginning to reconnect and regain his trust. Working with Mathew, I quickly discovered how to connect with him and stay connected to him during every second of the session. I used my voice in very calm tones, slow speech, and sang to him with descriptions of everything I would do; I also whistled to him. Whether he understood my words or language was not as important as him hearing the rhythms and tones in my voice, and how these related to the way I used my touch and hands to move him. When present, this type of contact created a meditative calm for both of us and for anyone else present in the room.

When Mathew felt safe, listened to, and heard completely, he would become accepting, extraordinarily calm, and relaxed, but at the same time awake and engaged. There was a fine line between a calm, engaged state and one which could change to being upset, withdrawn, and completely disengaged within a split second. This state of acceptance allowed me to find more and more directions of movement with him. We would work in a very comfortable chair with padding all around, which gave him a secure feeling. During the first few sessions, it was not clear whether Matthew understood anything of what I was saying. I was not sure whether he knew what a direction in space was or indeed the parts of his body, which I would say or sing to him whenever I intended to touch them. During the fifth session, it became evident that he understood me very well. It happened when I asked him to stop wringing his hands and put his hands on my shoulders. He did it very clearly. Next, I had him put his hands on the front of the armrests to make them long. I gently covered his hands with mine so that they would not slip and encouraged him to bring himself forward to sitting. After encouraging him a number of times, he went ahead and did it. It took some time, but when Matthew was provided with a safe place he could trust, he was no longer fearful. This allowed him to come out of his traumatized shell more often and for longer and longer periods of time. As the contact between us grew stronger, he would break into fits of joyful laughter and glee at what he was doing and how he was being related to. Matthew is a very good example of a child for whom complete contact, full attention, and absolute trust are the primary aspects needed before any kind of movement can be introduced. This way of working allowed him to sit more easily, begin to use his hands, crawl on his knees, and to come from sitting and eventually to standing and taking steps. Matthew was able to be present and move forward past his previous unpleasant experiences.

Individuality 8

Children with special needs or developmental delays particularly profit from individual adjustment of the developmental timeline. More important than the time at which an ability is acquired (the when) is the potential to make progress. This potential must be clearly defined, as must the path to achieving it (the what and the how). It is important not to wait too long with coming into the upright, with standing, and with walking, as these stimulate development of the skeleton, muscles, movement patterns, and neuronal networks, as well as improving self-esteem and understanding of the world. Adaptation of the musculoskeletal system to gravity leads to more efficient movement organization. Not only is it vital to appreciate and respect the child's individual particularities and consider using appropriate aids, but also their (familial) environment may not be ignored. All aspects must be approached with understanding and respect.

8.1 Adjusting timelines

Typical concerns: When a child visits for the first time, the parent will often say, 'My child is very far behind—she isn't rolling over yet,' 'He should be crawling by now,' or 'She ought to be sitting by her age.' They frequently express a strong concern, 'My child doesn't stand yet, when will she stand up?' or 'When will my child walk?' These are legitimate concerns. When considering the normative timeline of typically developing children, there is a particular 18- to 20-month period during which we observe the spectrum of developmental movement sequences and positions that ultimately lead to standing and walking. However, when observing and evaluating a

DOI: 10.4324/9781003737988-8

special needs child, many aspects of the developmental timeline need to be rethought and examined from a different perspective. This facilitates understanding of how to help the child to learn, develop, and grow. Becoming fixated upon trying to fit a special needs child's development into the timeline of a typically developing child only makes it harder to see the unique special needs of the child.

Creating individual developmental plans: In our culture, fitting into a timeline is more or less equivalent to meeting the deadline for a school project or at work. There is a clear set goal that must be arrived at in a fixed amount of time and must be presented for someone else to see. The closer the deadline, the greater the pressure; the further you are from finishing your project, the more stressful it becomes. Not only you but also those around you sense your stress; it begins to permeate everything. If the goal of the project is not met, there is failure: you feel that you are a failure! These failures often have consequences: you don't get the raise, the new job, or good grades at school.

To obtain a more fitting view of the developmental attributes of consistent spontaneous learning of special needs children, it is helpful to redefine the timelines. The timing of learning early abilities varies among all children, but this is even more true for special needs children with objective challenges. Each special needs child is unique, with their own rate of learning and acquisition of new abilities and skills. The direction of progress in the development of abilities is the same for all children, but the search for a suitable timeline is different for each special needs child. The goals and interests remain the same—a child who can learn, grow, and develop—but the path and timelines are undoubtedly unique.

Defining goals: To begin to re-define, re-evaluate, and re-calculate the timeline for a particular child, we must first understand what it is we want to accomplish and how we want to go about it. These two facets of what and how are important. They represent a vantage point from which to view and evaluate the progress desired and achieved. This progress may be in a completely new movement or element of a movement, in a completely new ability or skill, or in elements of the particular ability or skill. The progress may also be in the development of the sensation of a new skill or emotional/social ability that is emerging into the foreground. A clear and well-defined timeline shows us what needs to appear when on the spectrum of typical development. For a special needs child, the when and the how are not as clearly defined. All aspects of what, when, how, and for which child become factors in the timeline evaluation.

Finding the individual rhythm: For a special needs child, once something new appears and starts to form in a repetitive manner within a particular timeframe, the child can be said to be progressing developmentally. The progress needs to be consistent and clear. Once this becomes noticeable, it becomes possible to more clearly see a rhythmic appearance of new movements and elements of movement, as well as new behavioral patterns and social and emotional abilities. Each new movement, expression of emotion, and behavior helps to define the rate of the child's progress, which assists in developing a timeline for a particular child on the developmental progression scale.

Mindful readjustment of timelines for adults: Readjustment of timelines is also a relevant topic for an adult involved in a process of self-learning through movement. Adults present their 'problems' within a framework of wanting to be 'fixed.' They want it done quickly, and then they want to go back to how they were before. It is as if they bring themselves into a repair shop and deposit their body. Recognizing that processes of personal change take place over time on a very individual basis is important for letting go of a set idea of how something should 'get better' or 'heal.' Positive change and improvement as an adult can be a process of adjustment to a new situation. It can also be the realization that the 'difficulty' we think we have is a self-imposed way of moving or doing. For a variety of changes and progress to take place, one must be open to self-learning. Self-learning through movement requires mindful attention to oneself and an understanding of one's own way of doing, individual attitude, and ability to change. Some call this mindfulness or conscious awareness (Fogel, 2013; Hüther, 2006, 2018).

8.2 The importance of being in the upright

Advantages of an upright position: Watching a baby pull themself up to standing, then managing to stand on their own, cruise from one object to another, and finally take independent steps is a wonderful experience (Figure 8.1). The progressive development of the ability to stand and begin walking takes place after a long apprenticeship of many phases of movement over a time period of 10–18 months. This wondrous timeframe contains so many important aspects for the child's future development and relationship to the surrounding environment and social world. While all phases and stages seen before the child comes into the upright are important in themselves, being in the upright has many essential features that cannot be acquired, attained, or developed in any other position (Bainbridge-Cohen, 1994; Feldenkrais, 1981, 1949; Hadders-Algra & Carlberg, 2008).

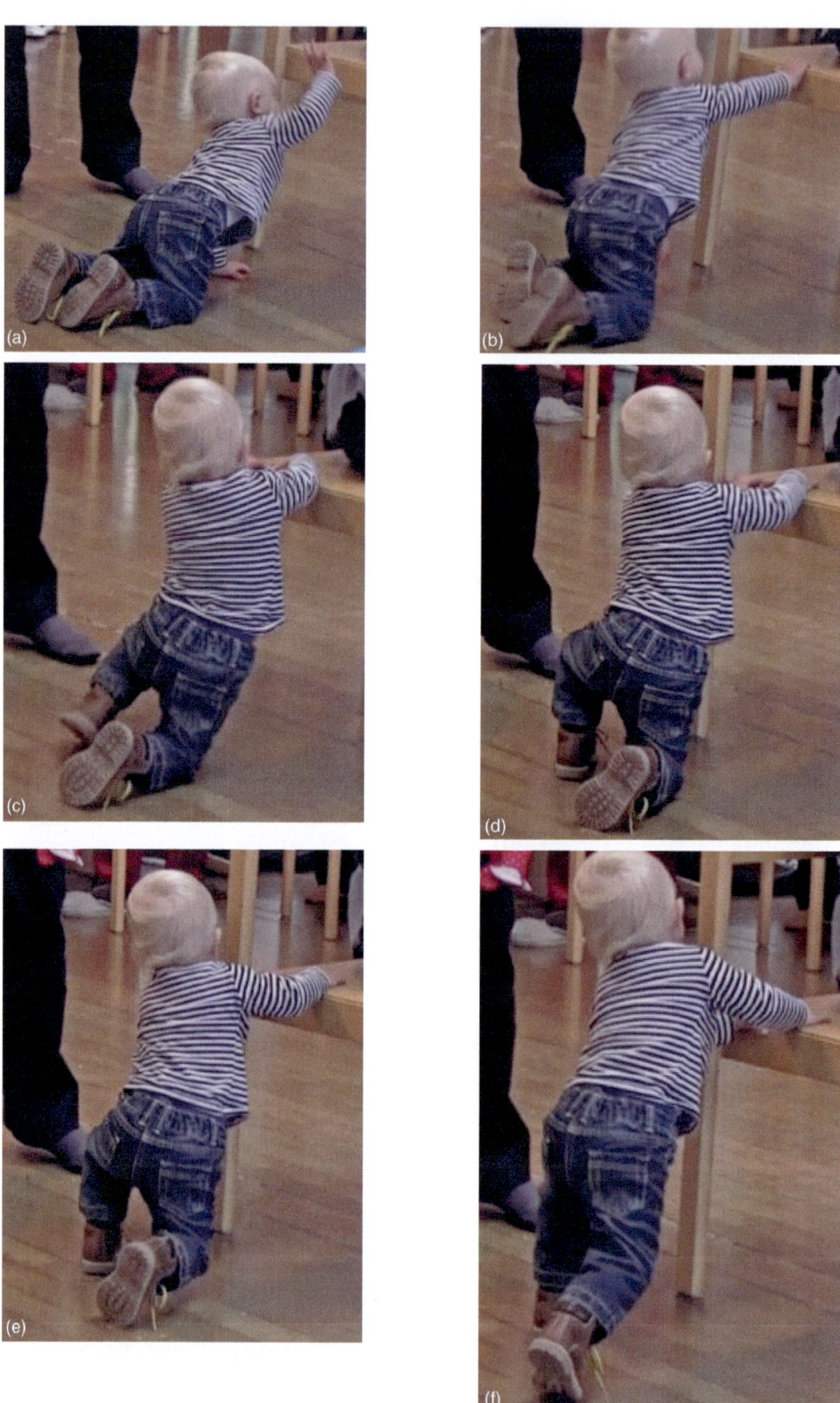

Figure 8.1: Coming up to standing

The benefits for the child of being in the upright are manifold:

- Seeing the world from a higher perspective: First and foremost, it gives the child a different visual field. The developmental period during which the infant starts off on their back with very few transitional movements and gradually continues until they come into the upright is a period during which the child's visual field and perspective become increasingly higher. Each successive phase gives the growing child a different, higher, and richer view of the world around them.
- Skeleton, muscles, and configuration: Being upright also helps to develop postural control and fosters continued growth and progress in the formation of the cervical (neck) and lumbar (lower back) curves of the spine. It is a vital part of the continued growth and development of the form of the hip joints, ankles, and feet. The weight-bearing effect of being in the upright position promotes better bone growth. This is complemented by using the muscles and also by configurations that are only possible in an upright position.

The correct point in time: For these reasons, it is important not to wait too long before bringing a child up to standing. For numerous different reasons, many special needs children do not find their own way to many kinds of movements in the developmental spectrum. There is no need to wait until a child does 'everything' that they are 'supposed' to do on the ground before bringing them up to standing. Being ready to be in the upright is determined by several factors. The child must have the strength and be able to push from their feet and legs to stand on their feet and stay there without collapsing. The age of the child is also very important. Waiting too long to get the child up onto their feet can be detrimental and even harmful for the child's future growth and development.

Arriving in the upright: In practical terms it is not always easy to bring a child onto their feet and into the upright in such a way that this furthers their development in the direction of independence. The skills needed to bring a special needs child into the upright must be learned, as they require an in-depth understanding of the organization of the body in the upright and the ways that are most helpful and necessary for coming into the position. Many special needs children have unique skeletal structures and muscular tonus, and it is essential to learn what to watch out for when bringing the child up, so that it fits for the individual. The sensation of supporting their own weight in an upright position is an important experience for the child to have. It gives them a better sense of Self. It is also very important for the entire musculoskeletal system to have the ground forces travel from the feet, through the hip joints and spine, to the head. It is important for breathing and digestion as well. It is of paramount importance to find the proper manner and time to bring a special needs child into the upright.

Standing and walking: Once the child is upright, the situation can be used to foster the development of taking steps and walking. The process of taking steps and walking is automatic. There are many ways to take steps and walk, and there is no limit to the scope for improvement of this ability. However, walking can only be achieved once the child is in the upright. The configuration and organization of standing and the movements that are possible in the upright cannot be accomplished in any other position. There is a thinking that a child must go through all the phases that typically precede standing before they can stand, that these are indeed necessary for standing. However, recent research has shown this reasoning to be untrue or not to hold up to reality. In my thinking, once a child has the strength and ability to push upwards and be on their feet, it is important to have them do so.

Integrate previous stages of movement development: Bringing the child into the upright does not in any way interfere with continuing to assist the child with improving its movement abilities and skills in other configurations and sequences on the floor, such as rolling, coming onto hands and knees, coming up to sitting, and crawling. It must be remembered that if all the elements required for standing and walking are part of all the previous movement stages, then it follows that these earlier stages are also being helped to form further during standing and walking. This actually allows for the typical flow of movement that we see in young children, who, during an hour's activity of play, will be on the ground in various situations, on their knees, sitting, and standing. In effect, by including—whenever possible—bringing the child into the upright, there is increased potential for better formation of patterns of movement, skeletal structures, and neural networks that combine all the phases and stages of movement development.

The series of photos in Figure 8.1 provides the opportunity to observe a child moving from being on hands and knees to lifting themself toward standing. It demonstrates an overall coordination and organization of the child's head, arms, hip joints, pelvis, and feet. There are many ways for a child to find their way into the upright and onto their feet. In these photos, we see a way with a clear view of how the child finds support, transfers their weight, and brings themself up from the floor in the direction of being upright on both feet.

In photo a), the child is supported on one hand and both knees, reaching up to the chair in front with the other hand. As they do so, the head shifts over to the left, and the weight comes off the right hand and arm.

In photo b), the right arm extends as the child brings their left knee closer to the chair than the right and brings their pelvis forward and upward.

In photo c), the pelvis turns to the right. The weight of the pelvis is outside of the right hip joint and is more to the right than the right knee, with the right heel turning to the outside. As the weight of the pelvis is more to the right, the head and chest side-bend to the left, allowing the left knee to open to the left and the left foot to begin to lift off the floor.

In photo d), the pelvis comes directly over the right knee, and the tip of the right shoe comes into contact with the floor. The left knee comes directly over the left foot, while the head comes over the left side of the pelvis and hip joint.

In photo e), the right knee lifts directly off the floor while still positioned directly under the hip joint and pelvis, and the left knee remains directly over the left foot.

In photo f), the head comes more forward and to the left as the left knee straightens. The right knee lifts higher and goes further backward, helping to bring the child more into the upright.

8.3 Anti-gravitation adaptation deficiency behavior

Adapting to gravity: Gravity is a force that we live with for our entire lives. Reactions to gravity slowly become ingrained in our behavior, actions, and patterns of movement organization. We must constantly manage the effects of gravity when we move and act. Early periods of neuromusculoskeletal growth and development are simultaneous with learning how to adapt to the effects of the pull of the Earth (i.e., gravity). This is essential to being able to move around efficiently in our environment. All movements that change the position from being on the ground, such as lying on the back, side, or stomach, to coming up higher and higher until standing fully upright with both feet on the ground, require managing our musculoskeletal system to move at different heights in gravity.

Adaptation to gravity via the muscular and skeletal systems: The skeletal system works more or less efficiently against gravity, depending on the position it adopts in relation to gravity. The muscular system is what brings the skeleton into configurations that are either more or less efficient when we move and act. Constant adaptive behavior is required to correctly orchestrate the movements we need at any certain moment. In the nervous system, there are antigravity mechanisms specifically for this. 'Perfect' adaptation and organization in movement would mean having a continuous and constantly harmonious relationship to gravity in all movements, behavior, and actions (Feldenkrais, 1981, 1949, 1985).

Adaptation to gravity via the neuromuscular system: In a typically developing child, the neuromuscular system learns efficient adaptation to gravity during the developmental phases of the first few years of life. People often notice and are impressed by how easily and smoothly a young child can move, and imagine how wonderful it would be to feel and move like that again, with a sensation of lightness and ease.

At one time or another, adults also experience sensations of being lighter or heavier in their movements, of moving more smoothly, fluidly, or being in a flow. These are internal sensations that relate to the individual musculoskeletal organization, as the body mass obviously does not change from one movement to another. At other times, moving and performing activities is accompanied by sensations of difficulty and hard work. There are many factors that affect this sensation and one's ability to move with a greater sense of ease, lightness, and flow. The way in which we react to outside stimuli and our awareness of these reactions is key to understanding this.

Effect of emotions on the neuromuscular system: Many emotions we experience during our daily routines have an influence on our musculoskeletal organization and a great bearing on our sensation when in motion. Emotions in the spectrum of uncertainty, hesitation, anxiety, and stress have a negative impact on breathing, balance, and functioning of the entire neuromuscular system. These emotional triggers reduce the functions of the skeleton that keep us in the upright, and, over time, slip out of our direct perceptual field. A constant imbalance develops between different muscle groups, and less efficient ways of moving become ingrained. These imbalances develop into adaptive patterns of behavior including sensations, emotions, and movements, which eventually become the individual's normative sensations of movement in the gravitational field. I have come to call this phenomenon *anti-gravitation adaptation deficiency behavior*.

Anti-gravitation adaptation deficiency behavior: These adaptive deficiency patterns are usually only noticed when beginning to feel discomfort, aches, or an inability to do things that used to be easy. There is an inner sense that movements are not as efficient as they could be and once were, and it seems more difficult to adapt to new situations in movement than it was. Understanding the mechanisms of how adaptation to gravity develops in the child's movements helps to appreciate how changes leading to a lack of ways to adapt our movements and actions can come about over time.

During the initial developmental phases, a special needs child does not have the opportunity to experience a spontaneous fluid adaptation of its movements to gravity on its own. In a sense, the child starts out with patterns of antigravity adaptation deficiency. The ability to compare sensations of ease or difficulty in movement, as a typically developing child or an adult does, is lacking; the path of spontaneously learning to adapt movements for ease and better flow is not available.

Developing a sense for movements and actions: The child needs an outside mediator to help them learn to sense distinctions in their movements and actions, to weigh the differences of one movement possibility against those of another, and to learn how to choose efficient paths of action for themself. In this way, the child will be able to develop the required neuromuscular patterns of motion for the most basic neuromusculoskeletal adaptations and make distinctions in sensation for smoother and more fluid patterns of action.

These actions may be as basic as lifting the head while lying on the stomach, or as advanced as coming up to sitting or standing. Once the fundamental abilities used and needed for better antigravitational adaptations are learned and experienced by a special needs child, they can continue to grow and develop. This paves the way for a continuous process of more adequate and competent movement adaptations becoming available to the special needs child (Feldenkrais, 1995, 1949).

8.4   Getting to know a child's individualities

Knowing a child's individualities: It is not uncommon for a special needs child to exhibit changes in the formation of parts of their skeleton and the ways in which they use their bodies while in motion. These changes can appear in areas such as the curves of the spine, the hip joints, ankles, feet, and bones of the arms, hands, or fingers. They may be ascribable to the different physiology of the child's muscles, to limited movement variations, or to a combination of these elements. Therefore, it is imperative to support the child in learning about their own unique structure and how to make the best use of it.

This goal can be reached by supporting the child's learning in a manner that enables them to recognize their specific skeletal and muscular differences. The child will need to learn how to sense these differences, so that they become recognizable and familiar during movement and while at rest. Once this has been achieved, the child can head in the direction of learning how to better control their movements and select a manner of movement more efficient for their own particular muscular physiology and structure. Sensation and movement go hand in hand. For some children, the sensory domain must first be brought into the foreground to foster a clearer understanding of their structure in motion. For others, the movement aspect needs to be prominent, because without this, the required sensory aspects will not be recognized by the child. This is something that has to be evaluated with each child individually; there is no fixed recipe. As the child progresses, develops, and grows, the particular learning direction must be re-evaluated.

Working with the child's individualities: A clear understanding of the typically developing musculoskeletal system is useful for helping a child to manage the terrain of their unique musculoskeletal development. Helping them to clarify how best to use their skeleton to fit their movement pattern organization also facilitates their adaptation to gravity. This clarification allows a special needs child to feel at home and at ease in their body. Once accomplished, it gives them better-defined access to their individual way of moving, without having to fit into a model that does not suit them. In turn, this eases the path toward continued learning and development of the fundamentals of self-variation in movement and movement pattern organization. At times, this is not an easy project. It implies giving up on the idea of 'standard' and 'normal,' of what 'should be' and how something 'should look.' The idea that each and every child has the need and possibility to move, in their own distinctive way and not according to a set model, can be a cause of great frustration and misunderstanding for parents, professionals, and, most importantly, for the child in question.

Consider using aids: It is sometimes not enough to use only movement and sensory learning to manage particular skeletal and muscular changes. They may need to be managed through useful and effective surgical interventions and/or by support from the outside to help with the positioning, structural organization, and change of muscle tone. Any significant change has an effect on the entire use of the Self. The better the child is able to understand themself in movement, the better the necessary interventions will help with the child's learning process.

8.5   Incorporating the familial constellation

Dynamic constellation: Each and every family is as unique as the individual people who comprise it. Its members and their distinctive personalities combine over time into a network of the behavioral interactions of the ins and outs and ups and downs of daily life. Each member of a family has a position and role in the family.

The role each family member plays must be able to continuously change and adapt to the altering dynamics of the family's life (Bowlby, 1969; Siegel & Hartzell, 2003; Schonkoff & Phillips, 2000). Some changes that take place are small and do not require a great deal of modification or adjustment. Other events in the life of a family require major change, adaptation, and adjustment. Certain changes are expected, and others take place over long periods of time. Others still are sudden and unexpected. One of these is the addition of a special needs child to a family.

The special needs child may be an only child, one of a number of children, the firstborn, middle, or youngest child. It may be a twin or an adopted child. The place a special needs child has in a family can be as varied as modern families tend to be. Whatever the composition of the family, whatever its structure, it develops over time into a dynamic constellation of its individual members.

Different needs: Each member of any kind of family has particular needs. The siblings of a special needs child play an important role in the family, and they also have needs that must be attended to and not overlooked. When meeting a special needs child for the first time, you don't only meet the child, but rather an entire family constellation. Being attentive to the behavior of the individuals as well as to the family as a whole is relevant to the success of the therapeutic learning of the child who has come to improve. It is particularly important to pay attention to the siblings. How do the parents relate to the siblings? Do they include them in the session? Do they introduce them with the same importance as the child who is brought for the session? Are they strict with the siblings, telling them not to interfere and that they should sit quietly while their brother or sister is being attended to? The behavior of the siblings and their responses to the situation are valuable to observe. Are they comfortable in the situation? Are they loud and disruptive, constantly demanding and drawing attention? Are they bored or do they sit quietly, reading a book or playing a game on a mobile phone? Working for any period of time with a child also implies forming relationships with each of the family members separately, as well as with the family as a whole. It is vital to intentionally give each sibling special attention, even if only briefly, as this has very positive effects on them and slowly but surely develops into an interested relationship.

Sibling relationships: Any sibling—whether younger or older—wants to be acknowledged for who they are, for their position and the role they play in the family constellation. The more they are welcomed into the situation, related to, and given attention, the better it is for their emotional growth and for the family as a whole.

A young child cannot cognitively comprehend the situation, why they are coming to such a place, who this person is, or what they are doing to their brother or sister and why. Often, they only understand that their brother or sister is getting special attention from someone. They see that their brother or sister is surrounded by great toys and is being encouraged to play with them, while they are being told to 'behave' and sit quietly, or else there may be unpleasant consequences later. Some of them are 'dragged' with the family from specialist to specialist for months and possibly years. Many parents do not really notice the emotional effects the situations have on their siblings. They think that because the child is 'normal' they can and should be able to handle themselves 'properly' and understand what the situation is all about and its importance. Or perhaps they are so stressed that they never really give the matter much thought. The parent may think innocently and without intent that the child should just behave and understand that their brother or sister is the one who needs the special help, assistance, and attention, day in and day out. It goes without saying that this is not the case in all families, but it is not uncommon and actually presents to a varying degree in the majority of families.

Depending on the age difference between the children, and whether they are the older or younger brother or sister or the twin, many siblings experience mixed emotions related to their special needs brother or sister. Some who have waited anxiously for their new sibling to be born and then wait and wait to speak and play with them go through a process of bereavement similar to that experienced upon the loss of a loved one or cherished pet when the reality is understood.

Before there is acceptance of their sister or brother for who they are, there may first be denial. After some time, the denial may turn to anger and only later to acceptance of the unique person their sister of bother is. In some cases, there is never acceptance. The siblings can often be left very alone and unseen with their feelings, as the parents struggle with their own emotions and the objective challenges of constantly managing all the requirements and demands of a special needs child.

The sibling may feel guilty about harboring such feelings and deny to themselves—whether knowingly or not—that they have such emotions. It may be that they try to learn not to be an extra burden on the family, as they are the child who is 'okay.' They may put themselves in second place. At the same time, they may have conflicting feelings, both positive and negative, toward the family as a whole or their sibling. Why am I in this family? Why has this happened to me? Why can't we just be like other families? None of my friends have a family like this. Embarrassment is frequently very present for these children. Having to feel, deal with, and manage such emotions from very early on in life can present both a challenge for the child and/or represent a concealed gift. Many of these children grow to be very supportive, concerned, and extraordinarily loving sisters and brothers, who come to appreciate the uniqueness of themselves, their special needs sibling, and their family. Others can become very bitter and resentful. There are many factors that contribute to this.

In the day-to-day work with families, siblings can be seen struggling and trying to express themselves and their needs. This can be easily observed by the way they behave in the situation, the type of attention they direct toward themselves, and the way they communicate with all present. It is vital to actively and intentionally give a distinct kind of attention to the sibling. This lets the sibling feel that there is someone who sees them for who they are, knows that they are also present, important, and deserving of attention, and that they want to be acknowledged. This attention may be verbal or nonverbal.

Siblings often become a central figure in the life of their special needs sister or brother in later years. They need to be nourished in positive ways early on in life and in a continuous manner. This increases the chance that they will be closer and more helpful to their special needs brother or sister and parents as everyone gets older.

Support and counsel: After getting to know a family for a period of time and having been able to show clear and continuous positive developmental progress with their child, it can be useful to find nonintrusive, nonthreatening ways to advise the parents and give positive coaching regarding the observations of the siblings and the family. It can be very helpful to offer a simple explanation in a kind way, discussing that—later on in life—the siblings will become as important or even more important than the parents themselves in the life of their special needs child and that it is important that every family member is taken care of equally. The needs of each individual are very different and must be seen, understood, and respected. When the efforts in this direction have paid off for the family, there is always a noticeable positive change and an overall effect seen in the entire family constellation.

My time with Dr. Moshe Feldenkrais   9

Dr. Moshe Feldenkrais was born in 1904 in Eastern Europe. As a teenager, he traveled to Israel and worked for a time as one of the early builders of Tel Aviv. He returned to Europe to study at the Sorbonne and received a degree in mechanics and electrical engineering and a Doctor of Science (DSc). During the same period, he earned a black belt in judo and was chosen by the Japanese Minister of Education to create the first judo club in France. He fled to Great Britain during the war years, and with his scientific expertise, he worked with the British Admiralty on anti-submarine warfare. Throughout this wartime period, he continued recovering from a knee injury he had suffered as a teenager. During this process of healing and relearning, he developed a multidisciplinary approach using movement as a medium for personal learning and growth. The theory and its practice were very new and unique at that time in the mid-20th century.

Dr. Feldenkrais was a man of his time, with a creative mind and enthusiasm for helping others 'learn how to learn.' He continued to teach his work until the end of his life. His method and way of teaching had a very positive long-term impact on many people from a variety of fields, as well as on his students who went on to teach the method and the applications of his ideas. I happened to be one of these students and also had the privilege of spending time with him daily during the last years of his life at his home in Tel Aviv.

Being assured of success as well as clarity of thought, understanding, and practice are the kind of seeds that became implanted in my mind as a young man during the two years spent with Dr. Moshe Feldenkrais. Encouragement to develop new areas of work through one's own creative process and personal experience was not something that was at the forefront of my thinking at that time. However, when you are told something—repeatedly and in different

DOI: 10.4324/9781003737988-9

ways at different times—by someone who is formidable in their own field and has a large personal life experience, the ideas find their way to take hold in your subconscious mind. Many incidents that help to mold a person's future can only be seen in hindsight. Such was the case with the time I spent with Dr. Feldenkrais. For me, at first, he was the founder of a method I was studying, but with time, he became a mentor, teacher, and friend, from whom I learned and gleaned so much to carry me forward in life.

Even though this time is now over 45 years ago, distinct memories remain. Many are of discussions on wide-ranging topics from the sciences to art and music, to mundane yet intense debates of local and international politics. Others are of the private visits from many guests who would come from all over the world during the latter period of his life. People who were prominent in their fields of science, medicine, music, dance, art, and politics would come for a coffee, a meal, or for advice and consultation regarding issues of both a personal and professional nature.

After guests had left, he would ask me my opinion of them—of their thinking, ideas, and ways of discussing, or even how they presented a topic and their point of view. The manner in which he questioned me seemed not to be aimed at learning my personal opinion of another person, but rather at prodding me into observing a guest's way of thinking about the ideas they had discussed. He seemed to want to find out whether I could observe, pick up on, and figure out how any of the guests put together their own ideas and presented themselves and their perspectives. After I had tried unsuccessfully to answer, he would then analyze all of the guests at length, in extraordinary detail and with deep insight. Why he was taking such interest and indeed such time to do this with me—and why in such haste after the guests' departure—was perplexing at first, and only became clearer later on, when some of the guests would visit again. The same questioning and conversing would commence anew once they had left the apartment. Yet this time, he would question me very directly about whether the attributes of the person that he had pointed out to me after the previous visit were now evident and observable. This was his way of teaching me the particulars of human behavior that I had no way of accessing on my own. He would remark on and analyze their movements, their manner of behaving and communicating, their motivations, and the weak and strong points in their work or relationships. He often would talk to me about the same person in a variety of ways, seeing if I was catching on to what he was so specifically pointing out to me. He would want to know if I could clearly observe whether they presented themselves with a façade or tried to discuss ideas with him that they really had no clear grasp of. It seemed so personal, like an X-ray view of a person. At times, it was so razor clear that it was uncomfortable for me to be discussing people in such a manner. I was only 22 at the time, and he was 78.

After a period of time during which this would repeat itself, I had the feeling that he wanted to initiate me, and mentor me in a manner of observing that which is 'deeper,' 'hidden,' and seemingly not so obvious. When he spoke about this, he said that for him, it was all very obvious, like picking something up that was just lying around. It almost felt that it was like a game or a pastime for him. He would often predict the person's movements, behavior, and reactions and responses in certain situations, and it seemed that he would sometimes behave like an actor to construct situations in which to play around with these different aspects of people's movement and behavior. It was intriguing and gave tremendous insight into people, their movement, and behavior. As a young man, this left an indelible mark and had an influence that carried over into my teaching and working with others for many years.

The confidence he instilled in me regarding my own abilities in terms of observing others, and the way he would relate to me as a person and a teacher, is something that I, to this day, try to give to all those I teach and work with privately when I present my work. I felt that through all of the discussing and the questioning, Dr. Feldenkrais taught me about how to be clear and precise, structured and creative; to always see the person I am working with an optimistic eye and to impart to them their self-worth and ability to rely on themselves.

During this period, Dr Feldenkrais was still working privately and writing. The preparation of his workroom and the greeting and management of his clients were tasks given to me. Whether it was an adult or a child he was working with, Dr. Feldenkrais was in need of assistance. The talks of the sessions after the clients had left were always fascinatingly full of the details and specifics of what had been done; he would talk openly about the progress made and results achieved. The relationship and attitudes of the parents of children who would come seemed to be of special interest.

As time went on, I was also given the task of cataloging the archival material of his writings, such as lectures and books he had not yet completed or was in the midst of re-editing, including audio and video tapes of his teaching over many decades. The exposure to materials in Hebrew that were not available to my international colleagues was a privilege afforded to me because of my fluency in the language.

The archives of his work consisted of movement lessons and lectures across a wide assortment of topics in the movement sciences and psychology of personal human development for adults, or, as it is now referred to, interpersonal neurobiology. All the lessons were created with the use of clear biomechanical principles. Accompanying these biomechanical principles as foundations of the lessons were embedded systemic means, which were aimed at producing personal growth and change. This twofold basis of thinking to propel change in people and their use of themselves and their behavior is what, many years later, has come to be termed and understood as 'brain plasticity in movement, attention, and conscious awareness.'

This represented a distinct understanding that experiential learning through the use of movement as the medium can play a key and prominent role in achieving better function and use of the brain. The ideas of neuroplasticity and interpersonal neurobiology and their direct relationship to experience-dependent learning were not mainstream thinking at the time.

Becoming versed in these original 'academic' materials of his method was a unique opportunity to take advantage of. There was time to immerse myself in studying the thousands of hours of information with hundreds of unique movement lessons. It was an exceptional chance to acquire the knowledge and expertise needed to become proficient in this distinctive part of his work and thinking.

This developed into the knowledge base from which to further expand the ideas into creative and unique new materials. With this huge base of information and over 35 years of experience practicing and teaching this work, I began to create and develop my own material, work, and approach, which I now call the Jeremy Krauss Approach JKA. The methodology of Dr. Moshe Feldenkrais is used and is present in my work and thinking. The materials and pedagogy are new and have different applications.

At the personal level, Dr. Feldenkrais always related to people in a way that gave them the feeling of being an equal—full of ability, creativity, intelligence, and personal strength. A sense of there being no hierarchy in the relationship. It was a persistent feeling of being full of abilities. An overwhelming sensation of 'having already arrived.' There was never the impression of being younger, smaller, or less experienced or knowledgeable, no sense of being judged or tested. The rapport felt very natural, nothing out of the ordinary. Now, when looking back and reflecting on the time and experience, it really was very unusual and very out of the ordinary, as I was only in my early twenties at the time.

This feeling of 'who I am' has stayed with me and infiltrated my teaching, work, and private life. Some of the greatest learning that happens in life and teaching does not come from reading or absorbing written knowledge or watching someone practice their craft. It is something more organic, like the way a child absorbs mannerisms, language, culture, and emotional states from his parents, siblings, and other close family members and their culture.

It is nothing that can be directly taught; it comes as a Gestalt, an organized whole that you experience together when absorbed inside a particular environment with a particular group of people at a particular time.

My time with Dr. Feldenkrais was and is very precious to me. I was always attentive to the fact that it would be limited due to his age and slowly deteriorating health. Dr. Moshe Feldenkrais passed away peacefully on the evening of July 1, 1984.

Practical techniques 10

There are four techniques in the Jeremy Krauss Approach JKA (Table 10.1):

1. **JKA Sensory Active Movement:** Detailed sequential JKA developmental movement processes lessons.
2. **JKA Abilities Lessons in Movement:** Group movement lessons for classes with adults.
3. **JKA Developmental Hands-On:** One-to-one therapeutic learning sessions for children.
4. **JKA Functional Hands-On:** One-to-one therapeutic learning sessions for adults.

Table 10.1: The four techniques of the JKA

	Groups	**Individual**
Children		JKA Developmental Hands-On: Individual therapeutic learning sessions for children
Adults	JKA Abilities Lessons in Movement: Group movement lessons for classes with adults	JKA Functional Hands-On: Individual therapeutic learning sessions for adults
Adults and children	JKA Sensory Active Movement lessons: Detailed sequential JKA developmental movement processes	

DOI: 10.4324/9781003737988-10

10.1 JKA Sensory Active Movement

JKA Sensory Active Movement: Sensory Active Movement sequences are well-defined, specific developmental sequences of movement done for brief periods of time with small numbers of repetitions. The purpose of these sequences is to experience and develop a keen, specific, and recognizable kinesthetic sensation that comes about by doing specific movements in specific positions. The sensations that arise from the movements are very prominent, usually come clearly into the foreground of one's attention, and can be described in a few words. The sensations that become recognizable include round, long, wide, short, thick, stable, tall, heavy, light, flat, small, etc. The expression is in terms of a contrast to the situation beforehand, e.g., 'I feel taller/wider/rounder/lighter/heavier/flatter.' Sometimes the sensation is related to only one part or one side of the body, e.g., 'My right side feels rounder' or 'My right leg feels longer.'

Learning to differentiate physical sensations: Contrasts and differences in sensations are important for learning. Distinguishing these contrasts and differences between that which was sensed before and that which was sensed after a specific sequence of movement carried out in a particular way helps to enhance one's 'sensory kinesthetic vocabulary' repertoire. It gives an appreciation of how quickly the changes in the sensory aspect of neuromusculoskeletal organization can occur. These specific sequences and the clear, recognizable sensation that results from the specific movement itself are repeatable. The same specific movement will produce—time and time again—the same specific kinesthetic sensation. This aspect affords the opportunity to familiarize oneself with a specific sensation and be able to relate it to a particular sequence of oneself in movement.

It is important to experience a large variety of these sensorimotor experiences. These types of movements and the kinesthetic clarity gleaned through them are relevant tools which can be used in practical applications and function in both children and adults. Any new sensation that is clear leads to better body orientation and sense of the surrounding space.

Understanding the relationship between physical sensation and movement: As adults, we do not give a moment's thought to the fact that we move according to and with the sensory information of ourselves, and we expect our sensations and movements to be congruent. If at any moment in movement the sensation of what we intend to do is not congruent with that which actually happens, we immediately notice and adapt accordingly. It is a luxury to be able to depend day in and day out on a recognizable continuum of clear sensations and recognizable movements.

Imagine the opposite with a special needs child. That they do not have this continuum, but rather a continuous barrage of contradictions between their sensations, movements, motivations, and intentions. It is hard for them to clarify specific sensations on their own and to interpret the sensation of the movement they would like to do. Having the resource of the specific sensory active movement experiences and sequences in therapeutic learning situations brings about effective and useful outcomes in helping a child become clear about what sensations and specific movements go together.

When a special needs child senses something new in their body and movement for the very first time, it is a special moment for the child. The tool learned through a sensory active movement sequence helps in recognizing when this has taken place, what movement it emanated from, and what the accompanying sensation is. Recognizing that it has happened for the child and giving them a moment or two to take in, experience, and absorb the new sensation is an essential developmental therapeutic tool. It allows the child the time to sense their body and how it relates to where they now find themselves in space, thus fostering learning and development.

This moment of pausing for the child gives them a sign/signal that the sensation is something important for them to notice, to pay attention to, and listen to. The child needs to know that both sensation and movement are connected and significant. The more recognizable the sensation for the child, the easier it is for them to follow and use the new movement.

10.2   JKA Abilities Lessons in Movement JKA-ALM

JKA Abilities Lessons in Movement: JKA-ALM lessons are guided, experiential movement lessons that improve one's overall quality of functioning and movement abilities. The various ways one uses one's attention and internal observational skills are of prime importance in both the learning and the teaching of JKA-ALM. The lessons proceed in a variety of positions: on the back, side, stomach, hands and knees, in sitting, on a chair, on one knee and one foot, on both knees, and in standing.

Experiential movement discovery: The composition of a JKA-ALM lesson is structured and systematic. The lessons are constructed with particular themes and are designed to create changes in movement and sensation. The specific outcomes result in an overall enhancement in the use of one's Self. The lessons last anywhere between 25 and 50 minutes. There is a use of a large variety of movement combinations as well as functional movement patterns in an JKA-ALM session. Focus is placed on what elements of movement combine together, and outcomes can be predicted based on how particular elements of movement are combined together in a certain sequence. The sequences generate experiences that affect the entire body and promote a great understanding of one's individual way of moving. Fundamental combinations can be used in various ways to create small and larger sequences of functionally oriented movement. In different lessons, different parts and sections of the body are attended to, such as upper–middle–lower, right–left–center, diagonals, and proximal–distal. People have a mixture of sensory, emotional, and personal processing types of experiences. These experiences vary in their nature, character, and substance from one person to another. In JKA-ALM, people also report that they have an overall sense of being 'more connected to themselves' and often find personal meaning in the lessons and the aftereffects of the lessons. The kinesthetic aftereffects can be very specific or more general, and they often vary quite considerably between individuals. JKA-ALM sessions can be conducted in such a way that there is more emphasis placed on doing the movements in an exploratory manner.

This allows for a less stressful and more pleasant personal experience. The accent is not placed on a goal to arrive at or that which needs to be figured out or accomplished, and if there is a goal to arrive at, it can be left in the background to keep the focus on the overall process in the foreground of one's attention. JKA-ALM may also have a lesson structure that requires finding a way to adapt oneself to a very unusual direction and type of movement. This may require a very different organization of oneself during the movement, so that the pattern of movement that one is trying to arrive at is done in a manner that remains in the domain of comfort while moving.

There are many uses of the outcomes and effects of JKA Abilities Lessons in Movement. One learns how versatile the body is and that the way we do something sometimes has more of an effect than what it is that we are doing. Sometimes doing movements at varied speeds, from very slow to very fast, allows one to learn about the speed needed to move in a given situation. There are different strategies that help the experiential self-learning that JKA-ALM has to offer. Each provides a way to become more in touch with the personal internal sensory domain. The intent being that when the sensitivity is higher, there is more clarity regarding what is being done in the movement itself. This, in turn, affords a great opportunity to change aspects of the movement while it is being done and not afterwards.

- Moving at different speeds: finding your own rhythm and pace, ranging from slowly to quickly.
- Active use of one's attention: learning how to focus as well as how to divide and actively change and direct one's attention in multiple ways, such as alert, relaxed, selective, sustained, wide, specific, focused, divided, and more.

- Changing and using varied amounts of effort during a movement by learning how to sense how much effort is being used and how much is needed to accomplish the movement. This is used as a way to access seemingly unusual or difficult movements.
- Pauses: taking more pauses during a movement sequence to notice sensory changes after a particular movement has been done.
- Letting the goal arrive on its own: finding a way to go in the desired direction but not pushing to accomplish; to be not goal-oriented but staying in the moment with the movement and sensations that arise. Letting the goal arrive on its own.
- Using the entire Self: having all of oneself become engaged while moving; sensations, emotions, imagination, thinking.
- Not focusing on correct: finding the personal 'correct' way, not a correct way in which you think it needs to be done. Taking away 'what is not allowed' when doing a movement.
- Using imagery and directed imagination: these are part and parcel of one's attention field and are useful in creating changes in movement and developing better images of oneself in movements that are not familiar or are more complex and difficult to understand.

Using different types of attention: Sometimes going very slowly allows more time to notice diverse unnecessary things we are doing in the movement, such as holding our breath or stiffening a part of the body not connected to the movement itself. Going slowly can give us the opportunity to let go of, release, or inhibit these reactions. Moving quickly also has its uses. It can help with not paying attention to details, but having to combine all the elements as well as possible and 'just do it.'

Moving with different kinds of attention and the way the attention is used gives the direct experience that how we use our attention makes a very big difference both to the sensation we have while moving as well as to the overall kind of movement we can do and its sensory aftereffect. Using our attention in numerous ways by giving attention to parts of ourselves we had not considered requires an active mode in which there is intentional shifting of the attention. This itself is a way to create change in both the way the movement is done and in the sensation of the movement.

Learning to vary the effort: Learning how to change the amount of effort used while learning in movement has an effect on how sensitive we are to the specific effort we apply and need to do something. Learning to vary the amount of effort in ourselves and learning to change this according to the needs of the movement situation is an important result of participating in a JKA-ALM session. Great versatility begins to develop in the way one learns, guided by the subtle yet pleasant sensations of one's own movement and not searching for the supposed 'correct way.'

Through JKA-ALM, a better overall organization of movement has the possibility and opportunity to develop in an adult. The fully developed abilities of the adult Self have the possibility to improve. This helps as a guide to finding better and more efficient ways to move that fit one's needs and structure—whatever the age of the person.

10.3   JKA Developmental Hands-On DHO

JKA Developmental Hands-On DHO: JKA DHO lessons are one-to-one therapeutic sessions with children. They are relevant for a child during the developmental stages and until puberty. During this time, it is possible to create long-lasting change in the developmental trajectory of a child's abilities. They are interactive and use all developmental positions and transitions. The sessions take place on padded mats on the floor, on a height-adjustable therapeutic table, on a chair, in standing, and also in a walker in the standing position. There may be music or videos on a television screen. There may be singing or discussions with the child or the parent. The aim is for there to be progress in every session. The session can be held one or two times a day, for intensive periods of a number of successive days, or on single days a number of times a week. Explanations and clarifications with parents are part and parcel of a DHO session. Progress and development is noted, evaluated, and discussed.

JKA DHO is suitable for

- cerebral palsy,
- genetic spectrum disorders,
- autism spectrum disorders,
- brain injury,
- *in utero* stroke,
- global developmental delays,
- undiagnosed conditions, and
- Down's syndrome.

The sessions help with

- motor spasticity,
- hypotonicity,
- sensory disorders,
- coordination difficulties, and
- gross and fine neuromotor skills.

10.4   JKA Functional Hands-On FHO

JKA Functional Hands-On FHO: JKA FHO lessons are one-to-one therapeutic learning sessions for adults.

FHO differs from other methods that use the hands in that it views its subject as an entire entity. This occurs during the process of touching itself. The practitioner has learned to listen to others through his hands: not only can they perform impressive-looking manipulations on muscles and bones, but they can also sense—through their hands and their movements—the needs of the other in that exact moment. This requires great skill and expertise, but also a high degree of sensitivity toward oneself and others—not only in terms of deciding which special manipulation should be applied, which is obviously highly relevant, but also with which qualities the manipulation must be applied. As the saying goes: 'It's not what you say, it's how you say it.' For FHO, this can be adapted to 'It's not what you touch or move, it's how you touch or move it.' FHO uses touch as the medium, with movement as the message.

But how does this translate into practice? An FHO lesson takes between 30 minutes and 1 hour, depending on what needs doing and how much the student can absorb. FHO is applied either in a chair or on a specially designed table in different positions (on the back, side, stomach).

After carefully observing the student, the teacher begins by selecting a starting position into which the person is then brought. They then start to move the student in different movement sequences; sometimes several parts of the body are moved simultaneously, sometimes just a single body part. This continues until the objective of the lesson has been achieved.

FHO is suitable for everyone—we all have some function that we would like to improve. However, most people who come to FHO have some sort of complaint, and most have already tried many strategies aimed at relief, including medication, with little or no success.

JKA Functional Hands-On FHO is especially suitable for the following:

- back pain, neck pain,
- stress and overworking syndromes,
- stroke,
- adult cerebral palsy,
- Parkinson's disease,
- multiple sclerosis,
- temporomandibular joint (TMJ) syndrome,
- stiff shoulder,
- flatfeet,

- vertebral disc problems,
- scoliosis,
- knee problems,
- asthma,
- anxiety, and
- nervousness and inner tension.

Although the results reported by practitioners vary, they are well above average. Someone suffering from various types of stress or back issues can expect excellent relief; someone affected by stroke can achieve greatly improved freedom of movement, reduced tension, and better control. Even people with anxiety and nervous tension can experience relief and insight into the causes of their problems.

References

Bainbridge-Cohen, B. (1994). *Sensing, Feeling and Action. The Experimental Anatomy of Body-Mind Centering.* Berkeley: North Atlantic Books.

Bowlby, J. (1969). *Attachment and Loss (Vol 1. Attachment, Vol 2. Separation, Vol 3. Loss).* New York: Basic Books.

Çelik Alexander, Z. (2017). *Kinaesthetic Knowing.* Chicago: University of Chicago Press.

Cozolino, L. (2006). *The Neuroscience of Human Relationships.* New York: Norton.

Damasio, A. (2010). *Self Comes to Mind: Constructing the Conscious Brain.* New York: Pantheon Books.

De Waal, F. (2009). *The Age of Empathy: Nature's Lessons for a Kinder Society.* London: Souvenir Press.

Edelman, G. M. (2001). *The Brain.* New Jersey: Transaction Publisher.

Edelman, G. M. (2006). *Second Nature: Brain Science and Human Knowledge.* New Haven: Yale University Press.

Ellingsen, D. M., Leknes, S., Løseth, G., Wessberg, J., & Olausson, H. (2016). The Neurobiology Shaping Affective Touch: Expectation, Motivation, and Meaning in the Multisensory Context. *Frontiers in Psychology, 6,* 1986.

Feldenkrais, M. (1949). *Body and Mature Behavior.* London: Routledge/Kegan Paul.

Feldenkrais, M. (1972). *Awareness through Movement.* New York: Harper and Row.

Feldenkrais, M. (1977). *The Case of Nora.* New York: Harper and Row.

Feldenkrais, M. (1981). *The Elusive Obvious.* Redwood City, CA: Meta Publications.

Feldenkrais, M. (1985). *The Potent Self.* New York: Harper and Row.

Feldenkrais, M. (1995). *Der Weg zum reifen Selbst. Phänomene menschlichen Verhaltens (Kapitel "Das Körpermuster der Angst").* Paderborn: Junfermann.

Feynman, R. (1999). *The Pleasure of Finding Things Out.* New York: Basic Books.

Fogel, A. (2013). *Body Sense. The Sceince and Practice of Embodied Self-Awareness*. New York: Norton.

Frankl, V. E. (1959). *Mans's Search For Meaning*. London: Rider.

Gage, J. R., Schwartz, H., Koop, S. E., & Novacheck, T. F. (Eds.). (2009). *The Identifacation and Treatment of Gait Problems in Cerebral*. London: Palsy Mac Keith Press.

Hadders-Algra, M., & Carlberg, E. B. (2008). *Postural Control. A Key Issue in Developmental Disorders*. London: Mac Keith Press.

Hanson, N. (1958). *Pattern of Discovery*. New York: Cambridge University Press.

Heller, L. & LaPierre, A. (2012). *Healing Developmental Trauma*. Berkeley: North Atlantik Books.

Hüther, G. (2006). *The Compassionate Brain. How Empathy Creates Intelligence*. Boulder: Shambhala.

Hüther, G. (2018). *Co-creativity and Community*. Göttingen: Vandenhoeck and Ruprecht.

Hüther, G. (2023). Was ist Potenzialentfaltung? Accessed March 7, 2023 from www.akademiefuerpotentialentfaltung.org/wp-content/uploads/2016/04/Was-ist-eigentlich-Potentialentfaltung.pdf

Kleim, J. A., & Jones, T. A. (2008). Principles of Experience-Dependent Neural Plasticity: Implications for Rehabilitation After Brain Damage. *Journal of Speech, Language and Hearing Research, 51*(1), 225–239. doi:10.1044/1092-4388(2008/018)

Knapp, M., Hall, J., & Horgan, T. G. (2007). *Nonverbal Communication in Human Interaction*. Marceline: Wadsworth.

Konner, M. (2010). *The Evolution of Childhood*. Cambridge, MA: Harvard University Press.

Krauss, P. (1988). *Why Me? Coping with Grief, Loss, and Change*. London: Bantam.

Piek, J. (2006). *Infant Motor Development*. Champaign: Human Kinetics.

Rywerant, Y. (1983). *The Feldenkrais Method: Teaching by Handling*. New York: Harper & Row.

Schonkoff, J. & Phillips, D. A. (2000). *From Neurons to Neighborhoods*. Washington: National Academy Press.

Schore, A. N. (1994). *Affect Regulation the Origin of the Self*. New Jersey: Lawrence Erlbaum Associates.

Schore, A. N. (2012). *The Science of The Art of Psychotherapy*. New York: Norton.

Schore, A. N. (2019). *Right Brain Psychotherapy*. New York: Norton.

Siegel, D. J. (1999). *The Developing Mind*. New York: The Guilford Press.

Siegel, D. J. (2007). *The Mindful Brain*. New York: Norton.

Siegel, D. J., & Hartzell, M. (2003). *Parenting from the Inside Out*. London: Jeremy Tarcher-Penguin.

Stergiou, N., & Decker, L. M. (October 2011). Human Movement Variability, Nonlinear Dynamics, and Pathology: Is There a Connection? *Hum Mov Sci, 30*(5), 869–888. doi:10.1016/j.humov.2011.06.002

Stern, D. N. (1985). *The Interpersonal World of the Infant*. New York: Basic Books

Stern, D. N. (2004). *The Present Moment in Psychotherapy and Everyday Life*. New York: Norton.

Thelen, E., & Smith, L. A. (1993). *A Dynamic Systems Approach to development – Applications*. Cambridge / London: MIT Press.

Thelen, E., & Smith, L. A. (1994). *Dynamic Systems Approach to the Development of Cognition and Action*. Cambridge / London: MIT Press.

Van der Kolk, B. (2012). *The Body Keeps the Score: Brain, Mind, and Body in the Healing of Trauma*. New York / London: Penguin.

Further reading

Carter, S., Maunder, R. & Laura, S. (2019). *Developmental Transitions*. London: Routledge.

Cozolino, L. (2002). *The Neuroscience of Psychotherapy*. New York: Norton.

Grandin, T. (2011). *The Way I See It*. Arlington: Future Horizons.

Levine, P. A. (1997). *Waking the Tiger*. Berkeley: North Atlantic Books.

Mukherjee, S. (2016). *The Gene*. London: Vintage–Penguin Random House.

Schore, A. N. (2019). *The Development of the Unconscious Mind*. New York: Norton.

Siegel, D. J, & Bryson, T. P. (2012). *The Whole Brain Child: 12 Revolutionary Strategies to Nurture Your Child's Developing Mind*. New York: Bantam.

Stern, D. N. (1990). *The Diary of a Baby*. New York: Basic Books.

Sundberg, M., & Partington, J. W. (1998). *Teaching Language to Children with Autism and Other Developmental Disabilities*. Concord: AVB Press.

Index